# Restoring Balance

**MICHAEL K CLIFFORD**
Rio Rancho, New Mexico

FDA Disclaimer
The information presented in this book has not been evaluated by the FDA. This information is not intended to diagnose, treat, cure, or prevent any disease.

I dedicate this book to Audrie Clifford. Because of her—as mother, supporter, and careful editor—I am able to keep writing despite being on the road. Thank you, mom, from the bottom of my heart for being there for me.

"Zen Stones" Cover photo by My Good Images from Shutterstock.com

Copyright 2018 by Michael K. Clifford
ISBN-13: 978-1719024754

All rights reserved. No part of this book may be reproduced or utilized in any form or by any means, electronic or mechanical, including photocopying, recording, or by any information storage and retrieval system, without permission, in writing, from the author.

MICHAEL K. CLIFFORD

# Restoring Balance

# Contents

**PART 1** ......................................................................................... 1
    Introduction ................................................................................ 2
Chapter 1 ........................................................................................ 4
    An Overview .............................................................................. 4
    First Things First: Qi ................................................................. 7
    Organ Systems ......................................................................... 12
    Blood ........................................................................................ 14
Chapter 2 ...................................................................................... 15
    Diagnosis .................................................................................. 15
    The Language of Diagnosis .................................................... 15
    Tongue ..................................................................................... 18
    Pulses ....................................................................................... 20
    Methods of Diagnosis ............................................................. 24
Chapter 3 ...................................................................................... 25
    Putting it all together .............................................................. 25
    Patterns .................................................................................... 25
**PART 2** ....................................................................................... 31
Chapter 4 ...................................................................................... 32
    Meridians and Points .............................................................. 32
    The Invisible Rivers of Energy Within ................................. 32
    Blogposts explained ................................................................ 37
Chapter 5 ...................................................................................... 38
    Types of Treatments ............................................................... 38
    Right Thinking ........................................................................ 39
    Right Eating ............................................................................ 40
    Right Exercise ........................................................................ 40
    Diet ........................................................................................... 41
Chapter 6 ...................................................................................... 55
    Body Work ~ Tui Na .............................................................. 55
    Acupuncture/Needle Work ..................................................... 57
    Auricular Treatments .............................................................. 65
Chapter 7 ...................................................................................... 69
    Herbal Treatments .................................................................. 69
    Duration of Treatments .......................................................... 78
Chapter 8 ...................................................................................... 83
    Cycles ...................................................................................... 85
    Freezing Wind ........................................................................ 89
Chapter 9 ...................................................................................... 91
    Organ Systems ........................................................................ 91
    Lungs/Large Intestines ........................................................... 92

    Stomach/Spleen ............................................................. 96
    Heart / Small Intestine ................................................ 102
    Kidney / Urinary Bladder ........................................... 110
    Pericardium / San Jiao ............................................... 136
    Liver / Gallbladder ..................................................... 121
Chapter 10 ............................................................................. 133
    "Got Fire?" ................................................................... 133
Chapter 11 ............................................................................. 137
    "You Be Damp!" .......................................................... 137
**PART FOUR** ...................................................................... 139
Chapter 12 ............................................................................. 140
    "We Don't Treat Disease!" ......................................... 140
    A Story that should have been a BlogPost ............... 147
Chapter 13 ............................................................................. 149
    Balance and Perseverance ......................................... 149
Chapter 14 ............................................................................. 153
    The Spirits Within ...................................................... 153
Chapter 15 ............................................................................. 161
    Women's Health ......................................................... 161
    Men's Health ............................................................... 167
Chapter 16 ............................................................................. 171
    Internal Causes of "Dis-ease" .................................... 171
Chapter 17 ............................................................................. 177
    Closing Thoughts ........................................................ 177
    "Wellness-centered way of living." ........................... 180
Recommended Reading List .............................................. 189
Glossary ................................................................................ 191

# Part One

# Introduction

My introduction to Oriental Medicine came through my long-time martial arts teacher. One afternoon while running across a street, I sprained my ankle. I was expecting to go to class that night and train; instead, when my instructor looked at my ankle, he said, "You waited too long. Now go home and come see me tomorrow afternoon. I will treat you then." I went home and overnight my ankle continued to swell. By class time it was the size of a grapefruit and very tender. My instructor looked at my ankle and had me roll my pant leg up to just above my knee. He then proceeded to stick six or eight needles in my ankle and leg. I did not feel anything, but the swelling reduced as I watched! After about fifteen minutes, he came back in the office and removed the needles. He poked and prodded my ankle for a minute or two then told me to stand up. Next he told me to do some jumping jacks. After that he said, "Go train." I was very impressed with this, as anyone would be, and it got me thinking about acupuncture for the first time.

I have always been interested in martial arts, and I trained very, very hard for over 20 years in various hard styles of martial arts, eventually earning my 4th degree Black Belt in the Korean Martial Art "Tukong Moosul." I remember one evening when my instructor said, "It is very easy to hurt someone, but it is very hard to find a way to help him or her heal." In the Oriental paradigm, the martial arts and the healing arts co-exist and are frequently studied together. If you look at the root of this, you will find that both are concerned with preserving and extending life; even though they may appear to have diametrically different approaches. It also makes pragmatic sense; if you are going to be kicking, punching, throwing and generally beating on your training partner, accidents happen and he or she might get hurt. It would be a good thing if you were able to help them after you hurt them.

My martial arts training as well as many other life experiences eventually led me to explore Acupuncture and Oriental Medicine. I attended Southwest Acupuncture College in Albuquerque, New Mexico earning my Master of Science in Oriental Medicine degree in 2000. In 2005 I had the opportunity to start teaching acupuncture at Asian Institute of Medical Studies in Tucson, Arizona. I wanted the opportunity to teach as I had learned from my time teaching martial arts that the best way to learn something is to teach it. In the fall of 2007 I stopped teaching and returned to New Mexico to be with my fiancée and to get married.

I am still a member of the National Endometriosis Research Center, as their 'Alternative Medical Adviser'. In my work reaching out to the general public I became aware of how little the average person knows about Oriental Medicine. It is to fill this void that I am writing this book. I hope you find it useful, informative and fun. I know I did when I was writing it.

Thanks,
Michael

# Chapter 1

# An Overview

I want you to begin considering Oriental Medicine by giving you a very general overview of the concept of health as understood by Oriental Medical practitioners. But before we can go there we have to address the issue of different paradigms. One could say different languages and that would be true, but it is more complex than that and goes much deeper.

In the beginning ... No, wait, it was even before then. One of the first questions becomes how far back to go in starting a presentation about Oriental Medicine? I could arbitrarily start with talking about balance, which is very important but we need to go further back than that. So I could start with *Yin & Yang* but even before we could go there we need to talk about *Qi*. Aha, here is something we can grapple with. One analogy would be the concept of love; much has been written about it. You might agree with some things written about love (on some days), and you may find other explanations totally annoying. But no one has really 'captured' it. The same is true for the concept of *Qi*, but it does give us an excellent, although slippery, surface from which to launch our exploration. The point here is that it's an elusive concept, which we will soon explore in depth.

I decided to write about *Qi* first as a way to start to explore the difference in the way "Westerners" and "Orientals" look at the world. In our scientific model something has to be definable in specific terms before it is fully accepted. Our Western society has adopted a belief that our scientific system is the ONLY real system and that all others are, at best, Proto-Scientific Systems. Without even a noticeable hesitation, we discard other systems. Yet these other systems, in particular Chinese Medicine, have a documented history of over 3,500 years. (Even longer is commonly cited, but as a minimum, 3,500 years is documented.) This system is complete and has withstood the test of time. Each system has its own unique strengths and weaknesses, and while I am not saying the Oriental paradigm is 'the only,' or 'the best' system; I am saying it is highly evolved, broadly encompassing, intricate and holistic. The other issue one has to keep in mind is that Oriental Medicine is based very strongly on 'relationships.' How one part of the system (your body) interacts with the rest of the system (the rest of your body) is based on these relationships. If one part is 'out of balance' it will, by definition, affect all the other parts of the system.

In a discussion about paradigms I should probably include a brief, respectful description of what I mean by a Western paradigm of Allopathic medicine. I am referring to the concept that in order for something to be 'real' it has to be definable in concise terms. As examples, one could think of mass, temperature, qualities of hardness, or fluidity; terms to describe "how something behaves or acts." These are fine, and they do work for many, many things. After all, they were good enough for us to put a man on the moon and return him to earth safely many times.

But I also want to bring to the presentation the areas where this is limited. In particular, our medical understanding of the human body is more 'mechanical' than it is holistic. This working understanding has created a form of medicine that is based on treating symptoms and is only recently delving into looking for the root cause of the symptom. As an example if a person has digestive disorders one is frequently prescribed a medicine that treats that symptom, often causing other side effects and does not investigate what is causing the body to be out of balance in a way that is manifesting as digestive disorders. One only has to watch a few television commercials to see the evidence of this.

Describing this same medical paradigm another way, I would say that this form of medicine is based on Newtonian Physics, where it is thought that the universe and everything in it is a machine. This leads to a medicine that is based on a different set of the "3-Rs" than we grew up learning; these "3-R's" are reduce, remove or replace; which is a very limited way of interacting with and treating dis-ease.

Describing the concepts of Oriental Medicine using Western scientific terminology is limiting; so we have to expand our ways of thinking, talking, and describing concepts to a more complete level.

So bear with me as I attempt to describe a way of looking at your body that may be unfamiliar. Sometimes it may seem complex and other times it may seem simple. There will be words that you are not familiar with, but try to not let that disturb you. I will include a brief description when I introduce a new word/concept.

When I write about what appears to be a "Western biomedical organ" but the name starts with a Capital letter understand that I am writing about the Oriental Medical concept of that organ system. A heart is <u>not exactly the same</u> as a *Heart*.

## First Things First: Qi

I would be the first to admit I can get tangled up when I try to think and or rationally discuss the concept of *Qi*.

*Qi* is the dynamic vortex of energy that flows through and around the body. It is the energy of life, an energy that is not measurable at this time by any machine. *Qi* energy has been called everything from vital life-force to bio-medical energy.

Pain and or disease is the result of the blockage of the flow of *Qi*. The body work, needles and or herbs are utilized to restore the flow of that *Qi*; if the energy flow is restored the body will find its own natural return to health.

Let me back up about 20 years and tell you about a truly-hard-to-believe experience I had when I was living and training in Austin, Texas. One evening, my instructor, Wonik Yi, was preparing to give a demonstration in Dallas the next day at a Bruce Lee Memorial. Grandmaster Yi gathered all of us in the school and had us kneel or sit in a position where we could watch his demonstration. He had two pumice building blocks with ten-pound weights on top of them and a car "leaf spring" straddling from one block/weight to the other, with the curve of the spring to the top. At this time I was working as an auto mechanic, so I had some initial thoughts about this leaf spring when I saw it atop these blocks and weights.

Grandmaster Yi stood about one half pace behind this and told us, "If I cannot do this tonight I will not be able to do it tomorrow in front of a thousand people. Now, be quiet and watch."

He lifted his shirt sleeves as he focused his eyes on the leaf spring; and started moving his hands and arms as he was breathing very deeply. Then he took a very deep breath as his hands went in a circle up over his head and he stepped forward; with a very loud shout his hands came down simultaneously and broke the leaf spring in three equal pieces!!!

He stepped back and looked at his hands; no cuts or scratches at all. Within five minutes, I looked at the leaf springs. As a former mechanic, machinist and welder, I would know if anything had been done to that steel by looking at it. There were no signs of anything having been done to this leaf spring; it was just a normally rusty, solid piece of spring steel. The breaks were clean and white. If I had not seen this with my own eyes I would NEVER have believed it. My expectation would have been broken bones, as you will experience if you ever try this.

What I was unaware of and/or unable to comprehend was that it was not his strength that he used to break the leaf spring; it was his *Qi*. Any human's physical arm strength is not going to be able to break an inch and a half wide by a quarter-inch thick piece of spring steel. We all know that. So what did happen?

What I understand to have happened in this demonstration was that Grandmaster Yi, who is the best martial artist I have ever seen, was able to focus his *Qi* in such a way that it was able to penetrate and/or break the steel of the leaf spring. But in this case it was his uninterrupted focus that protected his hands as they sliced through the leaf spring.

The next day in Dallas he did the same demonstration; with one significant discrepancy. Just as his hands went through the steel he told us later his thoughts "wavered" and one of the pieces of steel flipped up and nicked his wrist. Nothing serious at all, just a scratch that he said was to tell him "Pay Attention!"

So that is one example of *Qi* that is beyond the physical. There are numerous others, but there are many, many people that will swear that *Qi* does not exist, that it is nothing more than mind over matter or other limited and limiting definitions.

Another example would be when food is fresh it is said to have more *Qi* than after sitting overnight. Or food that is cooked in a microwave is said to have no *Qi*, or less than if the same food were slow cooked. The "life-force energy" of the fresh food dissipates as time goes by and the *Qi* of the food is destroyed or at the very least altered and damaged if it is cooked using microwave energy.

What we need to do here is agree that there is a life-force; that some people can control theirs better than others; and that this life-force can have many different attributes at any given time. This life-force is what I am referring to as "*Qi*." It is commonly pronounced as "CHEEE", though my Korean and Japanese friends spell it as "*Ki*" and pronounce it as "KEY." It does not matter how you pronounce it or spell it, but how you think about it will matter if you want to understand Oriental Medicine.

The Chinese character for *Qi* has two parts, the top represents vapor or steam, the bottom character represents uncooked rice. This indicates that *Qi* can be as dense as uncooked rice or as ethereal as steam. It also says that we get our *Qi* from foods. *Qi* can manifest in different ways but they all revolve around these simple concepts.

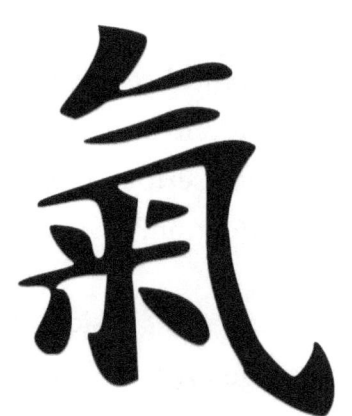

It should also be noted that in western science there is no machine as of yet that can measure *Qi*, or even detect its presence. This is what gives some basis to the argument that it does not exist; but I would counter with two points. First of all, it is extremely arrogant to say that just because our current level of technology cannot detect something that it does not, in fact, exist. That would be like saying just because a person cannot detect the higher levels of electromagnetic force from a television or computer screen with their own senses that EMFs do not exist. But wait, there are people that can detect and are affected by higher EMFs. I know this to be true; I am married to one of those persons. What about their experiences? Do we just ignore them because they do not fit our scientific model? Secondly, what about the thousands of years of empirical evidence that this system does work? I have always been of the opinion that just because I do not understand something does not mean it cannot be true. You can only guess how much trouble I had in trigonometry class when the instructor started talking about "imaginary numbers." I still get boggled by that, but they understand it and it was essential in the previously mentioned moon landings; even if I don't understand the concept. It works.

To be sure, there are some Allopathic diagnostic machines that can measure the amount of "energy' that is in a person, but it seems to be rather a quantified measurement of the electromagnetic force-field of the body. *Qi* is so much more than that. And to be honest, I hope it never is measured by a machine.

Some time ago, I had the pleasure of working on a woman that was experiencing a severe pain between the little toe and the next toe in her right foot. I needled some points on the *Gall Bladder Meridian* then went right to the painful area. When the needle got about ½ an inch into her foot, I felt a big "ball" of energy/tension. As I needled this ball of energy I felt it release. After ten minutes or so I took the needles out and then did some *Tui Na* (bodywork) on her foot. I saw her a week later and asked for a report. The pain was gone and she was back to running again.

The reason I write about it in here is I could feel the *Qi* as the needle approached it. It was like pushing in on a balloon with a pencil, springy and resilient. When I pulled the needle out, it felt like any other point needled. Once the obstruction had been resolved, the *Qi* flowed and the area returned to its normal state. No wonder I like this medicine, IT WORKS. Even if Western science does not fully understand it.

We will be discussing and thinking about *Qi* in various forms in this book, but for now I think this is enough.

## Organ Systems

When an Oriental Medicine (OM) Practitioner mentions your *Liver* or your *Heart*, *Kidneys*, *Spleen*, or whatever, it is important to understand that he or she does not mean your biomedical organ. It is a name given to a function of your body, much like the word "blue" is a name given to describe the color of the sky, but "blue" can also mean a feeling or emotional experience. So we do use the same word to describe very different things. For example if someone tends to 'discriminate' that could be operating from a preconceived set of values, but it is also the process of evaluating something in the present to determine its impact or value in a given context. If I discriminate against women or men or who or whatever in a given scenario, that is limiting my experience and the individual or scenario I am placing my preconceived ideas upon. However, if I look at a given scenario and attempt to determine the likely consequences of any choice, that, too, is called discrimination.

OM has observed that "Organ Systems" work in pairs; *Heart + Small Intestine*; *Stomach + Spleen*; or *Liver + Gallbladder* to name a few. This has been observed over thousands of years of empirical clinical experience. When one organ system is out of balance, it will cause the corresponding system of the pair to become out of balance.

One easy way to visualize this balance between pairs of systems is the *Yin/Yang* symbol. We see it complete within itself and balanced.

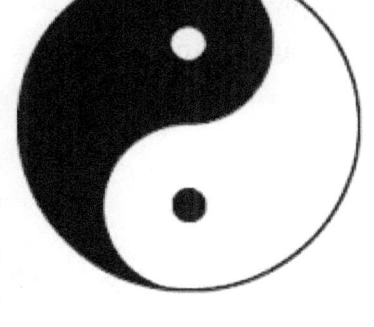

Notice what happens when one side is smaller (i.e. out of balance). It causes the corresponding side to be equally out of balance, though in this case in an opposite way, which is not always the case in our own Organ Systems.

Notice also how when the one side was drawn as smaller there was not a 'gap' in-between it and the other side; it is what is called a 'closed system' so any imbalance on one side will, by definition, be counterbalanced by the other side.

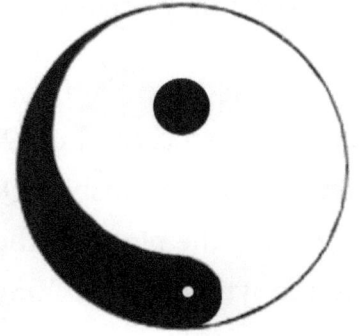

Also note in the *Yin Yang* symbol that within each one side there is a degree, or 'kernel' of the other within it. It is stated that there are "No absolutes" of *Yin* or *Yang*; or that within each is contained the beginning of the other. It is also understood that each side will turn into the other, *Yin* turns into *Yang*, and *Yang* turns into *Yin*. Or, as I am currently discovering, the *Yang* active, strong, vibrant aspect of my youth is turning into the *Yin* of getting older: enjoying quiet time, softer martial arts, and appreciating a slower pace of life.

In discussing Organ Systems, one aspect of the pair is deemed *Yang* and the other is *Yin*; one is deemed 'solid' and one is deemed 'hollow.' I will discuss each of the Organ Systems in their associated pairing and what they are understood to "do" in detail later, but we are still looking at First Things First.

## Blood

The Classics say that "*Blood* is more than, and not only, the 'red stuff.'" Don't you just love a statement like that? *Blood* is seen as the *Yin* aspect of the *Yang* energy of life. It is known as the substance that carries the life force or *Qi* within the body. OM understands that if a person loses too much blood they will die, but also that a deficiency of *Blood* has its own effects.

Blood is a very dense form of *Qi*; liquid, not ethereal, but *Qi* nonetheless. *Blood* and *Qi* have an intertwined relationship. *Qi* generates *Blood*; *Qi* moves the *Blood*; *Qi* holds the blood in the vessels, and *Blood* nourishes *Qi*. As with the symbol of *Yin-Yang* one cannot exist without the other.

# Chapter 2

# Diagnosis

One of the things I have always liked about acupuncture and Oriental medicine is the intricacy of arriving at a diagnosis. The art of the medicine has to meet the science in a way that is consistent, logical and straightforward.

One of the most common questions about acupuncture, aside from "Does it hurt?" is "How do you make a diagnosis?" That is a very good question, indeed.

I guess as a good place as any to start would be to break apart some myths and create a common language for us to use in the remainder of this book. First of all, as mentioned before, OM is based on a complete, holistic science. By this, I mean that each part of diagnosis or treatment is part of a whole, and that each part has to fit into the logic of the remainder. Ideally, the diagnosis will blend so smoothly into the treatment that you will not know when it changed.

So the diagnosis is actually based on very sound specific scientific criteria. Now the fun part comes in when you grapple with the fact that there are at least ten separate, functional ways of making a diagnosis. Each system is complete and when a practitioner has enough experience he/she can intertwine them quite seamlessly.

# The Language of Diagnosis

Here I want to open Pandora's Box and toss out a few words or concepts to contemplate. I feel it is important to consider that these definitions are "relative, not absolute" and will be somewhat different in context. But if we try to think of these terms as concepts and let them stew for a while when you run into them later they will not trip you up as easily. I hope.

One of the primary methods of diagnosis is to use the "8-Principles" so let's start there. This is four pairs of opposites. Again neither term is an absolute; it is a reference; or maybe you could think of it as 'more of this, less of that'. You decide. I sometimes think of it as a continuum with one term on one end and its opposite term on the other. Where the point is is the degree of the term. Does that make sense to you?

**Hot/Cold**: As you would guess this is fairly straightforward. There is either excess heat, as in running a temperature, or there is a lack of heat; as in one cannot get warm.

**Excess/Deficiency**: This, too, is somewhat straightforward, but there are some subtleties to be aware of. You can have both, and you will frequently find one caused by the other. To envision this look back at the "Out-of-balance *Yin-Yang*" symbol; can you understand how the 'excess' of one side causes the 'deficiency' of the other? Now many, many times the relative excess will be minimal and it will be hidden, but eventually if you keep digging it will appear.

**Internal/External**: Here we start to feel some complexity. Most of what "Western medicine" calls a disease starts off as an external condition. Think of the common cold. It starts off with aches and chills, sneezes, and maybe a headache. Without treatment, it will progress to a deeper level. It started as external and is progressing to internal; this is the normal progression of a condition. If it is not treated correctly, it will penetrate deeper and will increase in strength.

**Yin/Yang**: There is no simple way to put this, it is subtle and complex. The easiest way I have learned to think of it is the difference between a common cold which is a *Yang* condition, (fast acting, and sudden onset) and dementia which is a *Yin* condition, (very slow acting, and a much delayed onset). The cold hits you overnight, but dementia sneaks up on you and you may never even see it coming.

Those are the 8-Principles, and one can break any condition down to be described by these eight terms. But for more precision, we need a slightly larger set.

**Wind**: This is a great example of using what is observed in nature. Wind is said to arise quickly and change rapidly. It may be intermittent, and it may move from one area to another without rhyme or reason.

**Stagnation**: This is essentially the opposite of Wind. One old saying is "Where there is free-flow of *Qi*, there is no pain; where there is no free-flow of *Qi* there is pain". Stagnation can manifest in *Qi* or in *Blood*; and, of course, just to keep it simple, one can cause the other.

**Cold-Cool-Neutral-Warm-Hot-Fire**: I think of temperature in this continuum. This works for describing the condition, but not the cause.

# Tongue

In Oriental Medicine, the tongue shape, color, thickness and color of coating are all important. A very good practitioner can look at someone's tongue and feel their pulses and then be able to ask questions about the condition before even being told what is wrong.

As you can see, the tongue is divided into areas that are understood to correspond to Organ systems.

For general hygiene, it is normally a good idea to brush the top of your tongue. It does help remove toxins that are being excreted; <u>however,</u> on the day of your acupuncture treatment do not brush your tongue as it will remove the coating and will make accurate diagnosis harder.

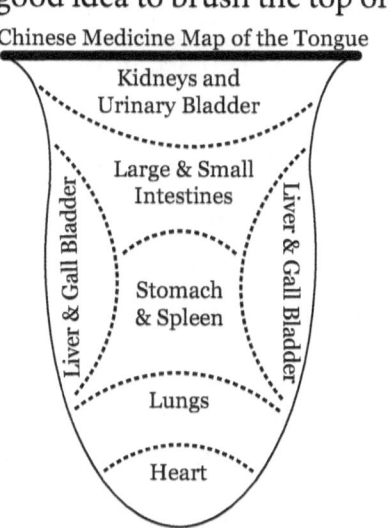
Chinese Medicine Map of the Tongue

When I was an intern at *Southwest Acupuncture College*, another intern's mother was at the end stages of life, and our clinic supervisor had asked the intern to describe her mother's tongue and pulses to us on a weekly basis.

For a few weeks, the mother's condition was staying the same or slowly deteriorating. Then one day the intern was very happy to she report that her mother's tongue coating had changed significantly. It had been a thick dark coating, what we would call a dirty brown phlegm coating. The supervisor listened carefully, then told the intern to get prepared as her mother was probably going to pass within a few days. The intern was completely shocked by this. But it came to be true in less than a week.

What I have learned since then is that this phenomenon is also known in western folklore; that many times as one is going through the natural process of dying, his or her body will seem to revitalize shortly before passing. I see this as the *Shen* making a final stand. I have also learned in hospice work that this is more common than one would suspect.

I consider this as another testament to the effectiveness of tongue diagnosis as an important part of the totality of diagnosis in Oriental Medicine. Even without seeing the intern's mother's tongue, the clinical supervisor was aware of the information that was there to be seen.

I also remember one day when I was supervising the student clinic and came into the room to check pulses and inspect tongues of the patients. After feeling the man's pulses I asked him to open his mouth and stick out his tongue. I was shocked by what I saw. He had a deep purple tongue body (*Blood Stagnation*) and a bright orange tongue coating. Very concerned, I looked at the student intern, who casually commented, "The patient and I already had that discussion." What he was referring to was the man had a condition that leaves a lot of sticky thick coating, but he also had an orange-flavored drink during lunch which totally discolored the coat. I wish I had had a camera for that one.

The tongue and pulse are used to check one another; there are times I would feel something in the pulse that would be confirmed by examining the tongue. But there were also times I would see something in the tongue only to be contradicted by what I felt in the pulse. That is when one has to develop insightful questions.

## Pulses

If you have never had your pulses examined by an acupuncturist, let's start by saying it is different.

When an OM practitioner feels your pulses she/he will be feeling the radial artery near your wrists, on both the right and left arms. The practitioner will feel the pulses for what seems like a very long time, but in actuality will only be 3 minutes or so. She/he will feel with three fingers on each arm and will be feeling at three separate depths. The practitioner has to have a very finely developed sense of feel in his/her fingertips that she/he will use to determine the 'quality' of the pulse. This is another area where some people may scoff and say it is impossible, but history teaches us it is not. This is one of the most important parts of diagnosis; it is truly an art form to behold. I have been extremely impressed with the level of accurate information I can capture from feeling someone's pulses.

Pulses are said to manifest due to the contraction of the *Qi* along the *Blood* vessel walls. To me this says that the *Qi* expands and contracts as it travels and this is consistent with spirals. If pulses are a manifestation of the *Qi* movement, it is vital to be able to "read" or understand what information there is within the pulse.

I am always amazed at the reactions I get when I feel a patient's pulses and then ask a question based on the information I have gathered. "Do you have trouble falling asleep?" "Do you find yourself short of breath?" "Do you have pain in your lower back or knees?" "How is your digestive system functioning?" These questions are relatively easy to come to from even a rudimentary ability to diagnose pulses according to the Chinese medical paradigm. I have heard of practitioners that are able to feel abnormalities that indicate brain tumors, or gynecological tumors. I do not have that ability yet; but I am working on developing it.

Another interesting reaction is from allopathic medical practitioners when I discuss the changes in the qualities of a pulse from one position to the next. The pulses are felt, primarily, on the radial artery just above the wrist. I think what gets hard for the allopaths to accept is when I say there is a substantial difference between the pulses when the pulses being felt are only a finger's width apart. One of the doctors told me "There cannot be any difference between them; they are on the same artery and only a quarter to a half an inch apart." So what I did was give him a quick explanation of how to feel the pulses according to TCM and let him feel the difference himself as I explained what the pulses were reflecting.

Each arm will have three pulse positions, and each position will have three 'levels' to the pulse. The right arm reflects the pulses (from wrist towards elbow, each one finger width apart) of the *Lungs/Large Intestine, Spleen/Stomach,* and *Kidney/ Urinary Bladder.* The left side reflects the pulses of the *Heart/ Small Intestine, Pericardium/ San Jiao* and *Kidney/Urinary Bladder.* I do understand the confusion when one feels a pulse that is closer to the heart, yet it is weaker than the next distal pulse. Part of that might be explained by the anatomical position of the radial artery. In this area the artery is changing depths from a position deeper in the musculature of the arm to one just under the surface of the skin. However a part of feeling the pulses is pushing deep enough to occlude, or cut off, the pulse. So, no matter how deep it is, the practitioner finds that depth and feels the pulse at that level. However, this anatomical explanation does not explain the difference in pulses felt by the practitioner. The only thing I can think of to explain this difference is the science of pulse diagnosis according to Traditional Chinese Medicine.

As mentioned earlier, it becomes very interesting to me to feel a patient's pulses and then ask questions based on those pulses. When I was attending Southwest Acupuncture College, in one clinic the primary form of information gathering was pulse diagnosis. The instructor kept emphasizing the importance of feeling the pulses and letting that be the guiding factor in arriving at a diagnosis. The questions asked had to be directed by the information gathered only from the pulses.

I know that I have a lot to learn and contemplate in the scientific art of pulse diagnosis, but it is always exciting and an honor to examine someone's pulses.

Some pulses you can't forget. I was giving a treatment to one of my elder patients and had spent a fair amount of time feeling his pulses, in particular I was feeling for any abnormality in the "*Heart*" pulse.

This gentleman has a 'heart-murmur' that is caused by mitral-valve prolapse (MVP). The mitral valve is what keeps the blood in one chamber of the heart before it gets pumped into a different chamber. When the valve "prolapses" it allows the blood to back-flush from the higher pressure chamber into the lower pressure chamber. When an allopathic doctor listens to your heart this is one of the key things they can pick up on. The heart will not have the famous "Lub-Dub" sound of the valve opening and closing completely. They say there is a "whoosh" noise that gets into the sound; maybe something like "Lub-Whoosh-Dub." I am sure that a cardiologist could explain and define the sounds much better than I just did, but you possibly can get the idea.

So I was feeling this gentleman's pulses and in particular 'listening' (through my fingers) for anything abnormal. I felt a strong, wide, slippery pulse; but what surprised me was I felt something "backing up" to the *Liver* position. In TCM we feel the pulses on the radial artery of each arm just above the wrist. Recall that the left side shows the *Heart, Liver, Kidney* pulses and the right side shows the *Lungs, Spleen, Kidney* pulses.

What I felt backing up to the *Liver* position remains in question. I might tell you that I was able to feel the mitral valve prolapse, but can I honestly say that as a fact? No, not as a statement of fact. I can say that I felt something 'different' and that it is something I have not felt on other pulses. Now I just need to be able to feel a thousand other individuals that have MVP and see if it is in fact an indicator.

## Methods of Diagnosis

**"10 Questions"**: More like 10,000 questions and in a paraphrase of Arlo Guthrie, "We will leave no part unquestioned". The art of questioning a patient evolves over time, of course. Where things are rich we tend to dig deeper, where there is nothing significant happening, move on. The initial questioning usually takes 45 minutes or so, depending on what is uncovered. I have had patients tell me "You know more about me than the OB/Gyn doc I have been seeing for over ten years". This is also a reflection of treating the whole person; therefore, we need to question all of the person, not just about the specific symptom that might need treatment.

**Looking, Listening, Smelling & Feeling** is also integral to accurate diagnosis. Your practitioner will be looking at your body, the color of your face, how you walk, how you sit and how you interact with her or him. He will also be listening not only to your words, but also to the quality of your voice and the emotions within the discussion. She or he will be aware of any peculiar smells emanating from you, and, yes, dis-ease does have a different smell than health and vibrancy. And of course, he or she will palpate any areas of concern, and very possibly your abdomen as well. From these four observations there is a great deal of information to be gathered and much of it will be subconscious on the part of your practitioner. It may be below his or her conscious awareness, but it is integrated into the diagnosis.

# Chapter 3

## Putting it all together

'Putting it all together' is where a practitioner has to take all the information gathered including the specific nature of the complaint, and her/his information from the pulses, the tongue, the 10-questions, and from palpation of the area (especially if your complaint is of a musculoskeletal nature) adding that to her/his knowledge and experience to come up with a diagnosis.

## Patterns

Here is where I have to break some "bad news." Oriental Medicine does not treat Disease. We treat Patterns of Dis-harmony. Doesn't it feel better just knowing that? Let's consider some examples.

John is 32 years old. Last night he was tired after work, and after dinner he took a shower and went to bed. This morning when he awakened he had a sore throat, and was feeling aches in his muscles. His wife felt his forehead and said he did not have a fever. That night when John came home he was very achy, he had a headache and he definitely had a fever.

OM would say that the day before John had probably overexerted himself which depleted his *Wei Qi* (Roughly corresponds to immune system) which allowed a *Wind-Cold* to penetrate (aches without fever); during the day that transformed to *Wind-Heat* as his *Wei Qi* started to combat the invading pathogen.

Sarah is 28 years old; for the last two years she has been experiencing strong to severe premenstrual syndrome (PMS). Her last three cycles have included strong emotional roller-coaster rides, and very painful cramps with her menses. She finds that she gets very angry over 'nothing' just before her menses, and after they are over she is not as easily angered.

OM would say Sarah has *Liver Qi Stagnation* that is contributing to her painful menses and PMS. She may also be developing *Blood Stagnation* but there is not enough information given to determine that for sure.

Cindy is 38, a mother of three. She has been exhausted since delivering her third child two years ago. She never seemed to bounce back after the delivery. She is now experiencing insomnia, forgetfulness and constant fatigue.

OM would say this is *Heart Blood Deficiency* causing her insomnia and forgetfulness. Her fatigue could be from overall *Blood Deficiency* or from *Spleen Qi Deficiency* not transforming the *Qi* from the food she is eating into *Qi* her body can utilize.

These three examples are extra simplified, but adequate to discuss the concept of patterns.

In the first example the pattern of *Wind-Cold* changing to *Wind-Heat* could be described this way: (John)

> **Wind**: because the pattern came on suddenly. He was fine when he went to sleep; just tired.
>
> **Cold**: because he did not have a noticeable fever in the morning.
>
> Changing to **Heat**: because by the time he came home after work his body had a fever from fighting the invading pathogen.

In the second simplified example (Sarah), the pattern was *Liver Qi Stagnation* and possibly *Blood Stagnation*. Here is a simple explanation.

***Liver Qi Stagnation***: Each Organ System has an "emotion" that is expressed through it. The emotion of the *Liver* is Anger and when a person has a 'hair-trigger temper' or is easily angered it is said that he/she has *Liver Qi Stagnation*.

**Blood Stagnation** because she is having painful menses she may be experiencing this pattern. One quick question I would have asked her is when she has these cramps does she put her hands on her abdomen and press, or would she scream if someone did that? This is an important distinction as it tells an OM practitioner if she has a pattern of deficiency; wanting to put her hands on her abdomen and press adds to the deficiency temporarily balancing it (in which case it is NOT *Blood Stagnation* but more likely *Blood Deficiency with Stagnation*), or excess where if she added to the abdomen by pressing in it would only get worse. Adding to an already existing excess is like pouring gasoline on a fire and wishing it would go out.

In the final example (Cindy) the simplified pattern was

**Heart-Blood Deficiency**: as we all know childbirth is a very draining experience; sometimes a woman will recover quickly and completely, sometimes she does not bounce back as quickly. Insomnia is seen as a pattern where the *Heart-Blood* is not sufficient to anchor, or secure, the Spirit at night; so the individual is restless, tossing and turning, maybe not even getting into deep sleep. But one does not usually see Heart-Blood Deficiency in isolation; by that I mean that it is usually a part of the larger pattern of *Blood* **Deficiency**.

Here is what I love about using patterns as the base of diagnosis: it tells us what we need to do to effectively treat the pattern.

Wind-Heat - Eliminate Wind, Clear Heat. By this I mean one would choose points that close the exterior "Wind Gates" and either points or herbs to clear heat.

Liver Qi Stagnation - Course the Liver, Rectify Qi & Calm the Spirit. Coursing the Liver is the OM term for moving the Liver Qi, or resolving the stagnation in the Liver Meridian. Calming the Spirit is about helping the Spirit or *Shen* return to its more natural and calm state.

Heart-Blood Deficiency - Nourish Heart-Blood, & Calm the Spirit. Nourishing Heart-Blood is approached through nutrition and herbs, and the nourishing of Heart-Blood will have an automatic effect of Calming the Spirit, and one would also choose points to facilitate this in the short-term.

Now isn't that simple? If it is hot we cool it, if it is stagnant we move it, if there is too much movement (Wind) we extinguish the Wind. I like simplicity, especially when it is so effective.

There is obviously much more to consider about Patterns of Disharmony; but in closing I will just mention the beauty of that name. We all recognize patterns; we seek them out in many ways.

When a pattern is harmonious it is said to be balanced, or one may say that it "flows." A natural pattern will seem harmonious in its surrounding environment. It is the same within our bodies. It is not natural to hurt, or to have digestive problems, or to only be able to sleep 2 hours a night; these are indicators' that something is not in harmony within our life.

# Part Two

# Chapter 4

# Meridians and Points

## The Invisible Rivers of Energy Within

One of the challenges to be faced is 'How do we wrap our minds around something that we cannot see or prove its existence with any of our Western scientific tools? At the same time it is being talked about as though it exists in the physical substrate.'

To be sure this is a difficult issue and it is one that causes many intelligent people to conclude that meridians are "Utter Hogwash." But I think we can find a way to grapple with this and then, having more information, you can form your own opinion; as I would want you to do with *everything*.

Part of the training one goes through in most if not all acupuncture schools will entail a visit to a "cadaver lab." Admittedly it was a challenge for me to go, but in retrospect I am very glad I did, for several reasons, but among them would be to see the respect these bodies were handled with at all times.

It was amazing to see the muscles, organs and nerves of the bodies. Each of us is truly an amazing creation.

But no matter how you look at a human body you will never be able to see a "meridian." Therefore you will never see an acupuncture point, yet they do exist. I use a word to describe them that has been overused, abused, and misused. It may even be a misuse in the way I use this word, but it makes sense to me. The word I am thinking of is 'metaphysical' by which I mean beyond physical, or beyond the level of 'Newtonian-physics'.

When I was teaching acupuncture techniques I would say that meridians "do not exist in the physical universe." By this I mean that as I said if you dissect a cadaver, no matter how deep you cut or what level of magnification you use you will not find a "meridian."

It is also true that you cannot see a "Spirit" or *Shen*, but you can tell when it is gone, like when a person is dead. You can also tell when a person's *Shen* is "twisted" as in severe mental-emotional imbalances.

The Life-Force, *Qi*, travels in discrete channels. These channels are the meridians. There are 14 major meridians, with inter-connecting 'tributaries' and a network of vessels. Each major meridian, except one pair, is "connected" to an Organ System, and to its "internally-externally paired Organ System." The exception to this is the meridians that run on your centerline in front and in back. Some schools of thought count this as one meridian, because they make one continuous loop if 'connected', and others count them as two separate meridians.

As stated before, the *Qi* circulates continuously through all of these meridians at all times, yet each meridian will have a 'peak time' when the energy is at its height and (for lack of a better description) a 'valley time" when the energy is at its lowest ebb. The peaks and valleys are 12 hours apart and it takes 24 hours for a full cycle of the *Qi* within all the meridians. But there is always *Qi* present in all of the meridians all of the time.

The *Qi* flows through each meridian in this sequence Lung > Large Intestine > Stomach > Spleen > Heart > Small Intestine > Urinary Bladder > Kidney > Pericardium > San Jiao > Gall Bladder > Liver back to Lung and repeating.

When I try to describe how acupuncture works I use this analogy. Let's see if it works for you. "Here in the Southwest we see a lot of empty riverbeds or arroyos. One thing that does happen when the summer storms come, is the debris in the arroyos will wash down to the next bridge. If there is enough water and enough debris it can wash out the bridge. I think of acupuncture, herbology or Tui Na (body work) as going in and removing the debris so that the water will flow."

Acupuncture points are specific places where the *Qi* tends to 'pool' or collect. There are over 360 distinct separate points not including the over 200 on each ear, and more points are being codified or accepted all the time. In general, points are located in muscles and not in joints though they may be right next to a joint. There are specific descriptions of where and how to find points, but even then it takes some degree of sensitivity to actually find the *exact* location of that point.

Stimulating an acupuncture point affects the flow of the *Qi* within the meridian. Depending on if one wants to tonify (build) *Qi* or disperse *Qi* one will stimulate the point (whether with Tui Na or acupuncture) in a different way.

Here is the clarification I promised about timing the insertion of a needle by my patient's breath. If I am "tonifying" I insert on inhalation, if I am dispersing I insert on exhalation. But even this rule is not set in stone. I can insert an acupuncture needle on exhalation (because the point tends to be less sensitive at that time) and still tonify energy by my needle manipulation of the needle.

I particularly like Kiko Matsumoto's choice of words as it reflects an understanding that "all fluids naturally move in spirals, at all times." As we have discussed, the dense form of *Qi* is Blood; and Blood being a liquid therefore travels in spirals within the arteries and veins. I see no reason to presume that *Qi* does not move in spirals as well. And that fits with my martial arts understanding of how *Qi* moves as well.

Each meridian will have "entry and exit" points where the *Qi* enters from the previous meridian or exits to the next meridian. Each meridian will penetrate the Organ system it is affiliated with as well as "spirally wrap" the Organ system it is paired with. Each acupuncture point will also have specific actions or the effects it is known to have; but it is well beyond the scope of this book to enter into that discussion.

I should also note that the actual acupuncture point is not a point as like the end of a pin. It is more like an area; some points are small, say the size of the plastic tube on a writing pen; other points may be as large as a quarter. Each point will be different, and each person will have a slightly different size within that range.

One last thing to contemplate about acupuncture points and meridians is that one does not even have to use a needle to affect the energy circulation within the meridian. This is called "invisible needling" and while not every acupuncturist would agree that it works, let me explain my experience and understanding of this.

Acupuncture is energy work; I think we can all agree on that much. The 'energy field' that is being affected by the acupuncture does extend beyond the skin level of the body. When an acupuncturist holds a needle above the skin of someone that is sensitive and in-tune with his or her body they can feel the energy being affected.

When I was teaching acupuncture techniques we would work with this in class. I would have the students hold a needle about 1/8 to ¼ of an inch above the surface of their partners skin and the partner would then try to identify if he/she was feeling anything at that location and if so what point was being activated. I found that the students that were more in tune with their body had a much easier time of feeling this, but nearly everyone was able to. When I treat my wife I can treat her very effectively in this manner. I can stimulate points and direct the *Qi* within her meridians without needling her directly.

My understanding of this is partially influenced by my understanding of quantum physics, in that as I understand that science it proclaims that everything is the 'field' and that matter is a reflection or form of energy, but that on one level even matter does not truly exist, so we can interact with matter (your body) on an energetic level (manipulating the field around your body).

Another level of this is from observing martial arts "Master's" that are able to do things that defy current level of understanding; like watching my instructor break solid spring steel with his hands.

There are things that happen that are not explained by "Western Science" yet they do occur.

## Blogposts explained

Here is one of the many posts from my blog 'peacefulmountainacupuncture.blogspot.com' I wrote in this blog for over 2 years, it was a way for me to express some of my thoughts and explore different aspects of acupuncture. I enjoyed the process, a lot. I hope you will visit my blog to see more of these writings.

BlogPost FRIDAY, OCTOBER 21, 2005
### Qi Knows
Last week I was treating a 37 y.o. female for chronic neck and shoulder pain and tension. She has had this tension for a couple of years and working as a food server for a living does not help it…
This was the second treatment I have given her; the first one helped a lot and she has not had the 'tingling' sensation running down her arms since then.

I was inserting the needles into the neck and shoulder area as part of a treatment protocol I picked up and modified earlier this year. When I put the needles into the area where most of her tension is located she asked me if I had put a needle in the outside of her left ankle area. I said "no, not yet. Why do you ask?" She told me that the area just below her left anklebone, on the outside of her foot was itching like crazy. I gave one of my usual replies, "Hmmm." I rubbed that point on her foot as I was thinking to myself, "now that is interesting."

One of the theories of treatment in acupuncture is 'local/distal.' In this model the acupuncturist will insert needles into the local area to release the tension, or blocked qi; then they will insert needles as far away from the local area as that meridian travels to give the qi a place to "go."

The point I was going to needle for the distal point was exactly where her ankle started itching. When I did needle it she commented that the itching stopped. H,mmm go figure.

The qi knows where I was going to direct it even before I got the needle in.

Posted by Michael Clifford, L. Ac.

# Chapter 5

# Types of Treatments

In ancient times it was believed that the more 'invasive' a treatment is (for the most part), the more the imbalance should have been caught earlier. The Ancients of Oriental Medicine believed that effective practitioners did not need to use invasive treatments. In other words, it might be said that if your doctor let you get sick, maybe you need to seek out a new doctor.

In fact in historical times, an acupuncturist was paid by everyone in his/her village as long as each of them was healthy. But when you got sick you did not have to pay her/him until you were well again. I like that; your practitioner has a definite interest in keeping you healthy.

They even had a different way of thinking about and approaching health care as we have come to expect. I think this is a very comprehensive and effective model of health care and I will be referring to it throughout the remainder of the book.

The entire paradigm of Oriental holistic living creates an entirely different way of evaluating life, health and the consequences of one's actions. I think this can be a very comprehensive and effective model of health care and I will refer back to these concepts throughout the remainder of the book.

## Right Thinking

It is currently understood and accepted since historical times that what one thinks absolutely affects your health. In modern times we have all seen this and instinctively know it is true. Then our "western conditioning" kicks in and we say, "No way, what I think cannot affect my health." Modern science is proving that what and how you think about your life is one of the primary factors in your health. One of the newest scientific medical paradigms is "*Psychoneuroimmunology*" or PNI which is the study of the interaction between psychological processes and the nervous and immune systems of the human body. (See Reference list)

## Right Eating

Nutrition is such a vital aspect of one's health that it is hard to overstate the importance of eating the correct foods. I understand that food is the most powerful form of medicine or poison you put in your body. Every one of us, me included, eat foods that are not good for us. Over time this will definitely have damaging effects on our health. To use a computer phrase: "Garbage in = Garbage out." In this case the garbage out manifests as poor health. I will be discussing diet in much greater detail below.

## Right Exercise

In earlier times, exercise was not an issue; we all had to work and work hard, just to get food on the table. The industrial revolution changed the amount and intensity of physical work one has to do on a daily basis. Some of us may even have lifestyles where the hardest thing you have to do is walk to your car. But this, too, has its negative consequences. I am not saying one has to be fanatical about exercise. It is more a matter of the correct type for your body type and age, the correct intensity for you and the correct frequency. I do recommend daily exercise, and I would include enough to 'break a sweat' every day if possible. I know that the more consistently I exercise the better I feel; even when I am stressed out and working a 12-hour day. One hour of exercise is more than worth the time it takes; my body and my brain always feel better after I finish.

# Diet

Now the first thing I should say here is I have only once met a lasagna I did not like. It was a strange occurrence in my life, but nonetheless, it did happen.

So what I am saying is I like to eat, I love good food, and yes, I have been known to toss back a beer or two or a glass of wine. The quality of food we eat, the way it has been grown, processed, and cooked is one of, if not *the*, most important decision we will be making, and we get to make this decision several times a day.

The Chinese historically ate 4+ times a day; they ate rice and vegetables and meat when they could get it. They ate smaller meals and ate more frequently.

Smaller, more frequent meals will jump-start your metabolism (your body's process of breaking down food into energy you can use). Your body also gets used to this schedule and if you change it quickly or drastically will let you know that it is unhappy, imbalanced and generally not as productive or powerful.

## Hunter – Gatherer Diet

I try to encourage what has been called a "Hunter-Gatherer's Diet" meaning if you can't hunt it, fish it and or pick it, you don't eat it. Now think of this for a minute. Meats, vegetables, very limited grains. NO processed food*s*. Or maybe think of it this way: a Cro-Magnon man or woman was not going to be able to go to McD's and get a quarter-pounder, or a chick-fillet sandwich from a chicken that has never seen dirt, or a cow that was fed all kinds of things we definitely do not want to know about (even though we need to). My point is that as we consume highly processed, or over processed food it does have a negative impact on our health. Minimally processed food will always be a better choice.

I will come back to this from a different angle after I cover a few other points.

**Balance and Variety**

One of the issues pertaining to our diet is that we do not have a good balance of proteins, fiber, good carbohydrates and essential fatty acids. When I was in acupuncture school, I found a great book that made a LOT of sense to me about dietary requirements. *Eat 4 YOUR Blood Type* (see reference list) had an idea I had not crossed before, but one that makes a very significant point.

The four blood types actually need a slightly different diet. The author, Dr. Peter J. DÁdamo, has made a career out of this research and has all kinds of studies to verify what he claims. His work may be controversial and I would encourage you to review both his claims and the counter-claims. [https://www.consumeraffairs.com/news/blood-type-diet-debunked-011614.html][1]

But his research works for me. At the time I read this book I was just dating the woman who became my wife. She had been a vegetarian for nearly a decade at that point, even though she would occasionally eat chicken or fish. Her blood type is type O, which according to this book needs to eat red meat. I got her to read the book, as I knew she would need to hear this information from someone other than her carnivorous boyfriend. It made a distinct impression and she allowed herself to modify her diet according to these guidelines. That made HUGE change in her energy, cognition and overall health. Now, more than a decade later, she is a regular meat eater and is much healthier for this change. She even admits what a huge difference this made in her life.

On the other hand I have type A blood, one that does not need to eat as much red meat, though occasionally if I am training really hard, I do need to consume more high protein red meat.

When I was teaching Oriental medicine and was asked about diet I would recommend this book. When the discussion came to vegetarianism, I confessed that I had a biased opinion and I know I still do. I look at the shape of our teeth; as I see it they are primarily meant for meat eating, not primarily vegetable or leaf eating. Additionally, unless one is extremely careful in their diet they will not get enough proteins, minerals and amino acids from a vegetarian diet. I know it may not be polite to say, but in my opinion some of the least healthy people I know are vegetarians. They do not seem to have the necessary information to be able to get the needed nutrients in the correct bio-available manner to allow their bodies to assimilate the nutrition they are consuming. It can be done, we all know that, but it does take diligent work. I will also have to admit that I do not believe diet is a matter of spiritual significance; that is a matter of internal discipline and attention.

It is well known that we need to get a good balance and variety in our diet. I think the more prevalent issue is that this type of diet requires preparation time, which is a very precious commodity in our society.

The time factor is a major reason why we choose to eat processed foods most of the time. It is asking a lot to ask someone to work, take care of the house and kids AND cook good quality foods. I know that, so I try to participate in this dance as well.

However, I would recommend a change in the way we approach this. Learn to make the cooking as much fun as you can, given the scenario at your home. If there is room in the kitchen, get some help. If there is less room, as there is in our kitchen, then share the cooking and cleaning so that neither one feels like they are carrying the full load.

It does not have to be a grueling, tedious chore. But as I keep saying: Food is the most powerful medicine or poison you put into your body. Make sure you understand the consequences of your choices.

Another very good nutritional book is *Healing with Whole Foods* by Paul Pitchford. (See Reference List) One of the things I like about his book is that it is a mix of Oriental medicine and some western science. He has some very good recipes and suggestions, though he is a vegetarian and does not eat red meat. Again I would ask you to read both books and make up your OWN mind. Both have very good information and I choose to combine the ideas of both (and a few other sources) into my dietary choices.

## Grains and the Industrial Revolution

When society started to develop agriculture, a few things started to happen that took a couple of thousand years before the consequences started to be realized in our genetic profile. We have been and are able to consume a limited amount of wheat, but as agriculture increased its ability to grow this food, our bodies have not been able to keep up (genetically) with the normal consumption.

In particular, I am referring to <u>glutens</u>; the protein in wheat, barley and rye. Many of us are unable to adequately process the gluten and our body has a distinct response to this as it causes inflammation, the subtle swelling of tissues primarily in your abdomen. Also be sure you understand that no matter what you may have heard before, you do not have to be diagnosed with "Celiac Disease" to have gluten intolerance.

Many people eat a relatively good diet, exercise regularly and still have an abdomen that is swollen or carrying excess weight. Frequently they will ask themselves, "What is going on?" Well one very good possibility is that their body is having a very slight, sub-clinical inflammatory response to the glutens. If they would remove all the glutens from their diet, (and I am not talking about just removing wheat --- you have to make a concerted effort to do this right, as wheat and glutens are hidden in many ingredient lists), I would be willing to bet that inside two weeks they would feel much better, think more clearly, and their joints would ache less. Additionally, they may be noticing their slacks and or blouse or shirt fit better.

When the processing of wheat into flour started to include chemicals, (in particular, <u>bromide)</u> something really bad started to happen. Not to get too technical on you, but this is important so please bear with me for this. Our body requires Iodine, as we all probably know, but bromide is in the same chemical family (halogens) and is nearly atomically identical to iodine. What this means is that when your body has bromide in the food you eat, nearly all wheat flours and much more, bromide will out-compete the Iodine for receptors. This drastically affects your thyroid, because the thyroid cannot process the bromide and the thyroid affects the metabolism and health of every cell in your body. So now because we are all being exposed to this chemical on a daily basis, our bodies are not getting the correct amount of Iodine and our thyroids are not functioning at full capability.

I am saying that even with the best of intentions, we are poisoning our bodies on a daily basis, and this is going to have health consequences whether we like it or not.

Another very similar sounding, yet different additive is Potassium Bromate which is added to wheat flour to strengthen it in the kneading process. Every industrialized country in the world EXCEPT THE UNITED STATES has banned this as a food additive since 1991 as it is a KNOWN CARCINOGEN. In the United States, it has not been banned.

The FDA sanctioned the use of bromate before the Delaney clause of the Food, Drug, and Cosmetic Act went into effect in 1958, which bans carcinogenic substances, so that it is more difficult for it to now be banned. Instead, since 1991 the FDA has urged bakers to voluntarily stop using it. In California, a warning label is required when bromated flour is used. Look at the flour in your cupboard or in a store to see if it says anything about this, or says non-bromated. Just because it does not say anything does not actually mean it is or is not brominated. To me, this is like seeing turn-signals flashing on a car; all that really means is the turn signals on that car work. Nothing more, nothing less.

This is a very significant indication that the FDA is not fulfilling its charter obligations and is allowing known carcinogens to potentially be in our food supply. This is unacceptable but unless we raise the issue it will remain in the background.

**Freshness and Source**

Also when our society started to migrate into towns to work in factories, our diet changed, in that the foods 'city dwellers' eat are usually not as fresh, and we are at least two or three steps removed from their growing and harvesting. I do feel this is an important piece of the equation.

I also think it is important to eat foods that are grown locally as much as possible. I try to not eat foods from South America or China; why you ask? Let me be clear, from my perspective it has nothing to do with the quality of their food; though that is impacted by the time it takes to ship the foods around the world or across the nation. From my perspective it is because the microorganisms those foods grew up with are not the same microorganisms that I have to deal with on a daily basis. My body (and yours) responds better to having one particular region's microorganism, and not a 'hodge-podge, mix and match session' created by humongous agribusiness industries.

Our immune systems apparently get some kind of information from the foods we are ingesting and use this food-information to be able to develop an immune response to potential pathogens. What do you think happens when they get information to respond to "microorganism F" but are actually exposed to "microorganism R"? It is like thinking my sparring partner is going to try a round-house kick which I am preparing to counter when actually he just punches me in the belly. Not only do I end up sucking air, but I hate it when that happens.

There is another reason why I try to buy locally as much as possible. That is because of the 'time-lag' of shipping the food across the ocean or country to my local store. Remember, freshness is an integral part of quality. Additionally the money I spend in a local farmer's market stays primarily within the community to circulate and help the community prosper as compared to a national chain that takes its money out the community and only pays wages and overhead for the store.

## Quantity and Quality

In general, nearly everyone I know eats too much food at one time; we wait too long between meals and then we eat fair-to-poor quality food when we do eat.

I grew up in the 1960's and the level of obesity then was what, a third as prevalent as it now? And when you look at the actual quality of the nutrients in the foods, you'll find they have a much lower nutritional value than the same food from 30+ years ago. There are many reasons for that, but as strange as it may seem, one of the primary causes is the types and amount of fertilizer being used.

Historically, farmers knew to let the ground lay 'fallow' for one out of every seven years. Just let it rest. Agribusiness does not want to do that, so they pump chemicals into the ground in order to make the plants grow. But it is a 'hollow' or 'empty' *Qi* within the food --- a food that has no true *Qi* to give. What will that do to your health over the length of your life? It is worth contemplating.

Again, I strongly recommend buying local foods at a farmer's market if at all possible, locating a good quality meat market and striving to get organic foods whenever possible. I know we can't always do that, but it is important to try to do this as much as possible.

We also all need to eat less; well, maybe not everyone, but the vast majority of us do.

## Quality of Cooking

Earlier, I mentioned that cooking food with a microwave oven damages or destroys the nutritional content of that food. I am going to explain that in more detail now.

There are actually two concerns about the quality of cooking one uses in preparing foods, both of these concerns are present, in degree, no matter how one cooks, but one is only present with microwave cooking.

First let me define microwave energy as used in cooking, it is a series of very high frequency electromagnetic waves of energy being focused into a substance which causes the water and fat in that substance to become "excited", or cause them to vibrate at a higher rate. This increased rate of vibration causes friction which causes heat. That is the cause of the concern as well.

By causing the liquids (water, fats or whatever) to be exposed to this very high frequency of radio waves (electromagnetic waves) it alters the *structure* of the substance. While it is true that any form of cooking alters the structure (proteins unravel for example) there is a difference in how this alteration occurs and the degree of the alteration.

Also a very serious concern is: what happens to any residual energy left in the foods?

As you know from touching a TV screen after it has been turned off, it takes TIME for that energy to dissipate. The energy in a TV screen is also electromagnetic, but of a different (much lower) level than microwave transmission and reception. Think of the cell-phone towers in our neighborhoods, they are capable of sending data as far as they can see in line of sight, and further, through the atmosphere. That kind of energy being pumped into our foods has got to have some kind of lasting effect. It does not just dissipate while you carry the food to the table (or couch) before you eat it.

What will be the effects of eating foods that have a degree of residual microwave energy still within them over a lifetime? Only our future generations will be able to tell, but it is a very reasonable bet to say there will be some consequence. There always is.

The other concern about the quality of cooking is overcooking the food, which reduces the nutritional content. As I mentioned earlier, protein 'unravels' when it is cooked. This can be a good thing, up to a point; but over-cooking proteins actually destroys the nutritional value of the food, no matter how it is cooked.

Carbohydrates have a similar, yet different issue in that the way that our body recognizes and thereby recovers the value of the carbohydrate is due to the shape of the carbohydrate. I think of it like a key that has to fit into a certain lock in order to unlock, or activate it. What happens if some of the notches on that key are bent, filed smooth or otherwise altered? The lock may or may not open as desired. Essential Fatty Acids (EFAs) are particularly susceptible to becoming misshapen due to heat. (Which is why it is important to get 'fish oils' that have been cold processed. If you can taste 'fish' or you belch it back up after swallowing it is rancid and by definition not a good quality.)

## A Quick Word on Herbs

It is important to understand that the Chinese in particular have been working with herbal remedies for thousands of years. In fact, their first written book was on herbology, not religion or commerce, philosophy or anything else. It was a systematic, concise book, complete with accurate drawings of all the plants and how they were to be used.

There are a couple of things I need to put in at this point. First of all, **DO NOT MAKE YOUR OWN HERBAL REMEDIES, POTIONS OR LOTIONS**, unless you have been trained in the correct and safe use of these herbs. Sometimes one may think "Oh, they are only herbs; they are not that powerful." Making your own herbal remedy would be a mistake, possibly a fatal one. Please understand this, I love herbs! I think they are very powerful medicine and if used correctly, will be of great assistance in returning one to a balanced state of health. I also know that if someone makes an incorrect diagnosis and uses the wrong herb combination it can be devastating.

My second point is that wherever you get your herbal remedies; make sure the supply company is using *clean, correctly processed herbs*. It is a beautiful mix between science and art to correctly grow, harvest and process Chinese herbs. Do not take anything without some polite but serious questions about source and processing. There are some *great* herbal supply companies in the U.S. which process herbs in clean, safe, secure facilities. Look in the Glossary, and ask your acupuncturist what company she/he uses.

**Supplements**

Admittedly, the nutritional value of the foods we eat is lower now than it was 30+ years ago. What this means is we need to supplement our nutrition with high quality supplements. (See Reference list) High quality supplements can help treat many, many concerns from digestive to musculoskeletal to emotional imbalances. But again I stress the word "high" quality; that is unless you like letting your hard-earned money get flushed down the toilet every day...

And make sure you understand this, you cannot just start taking supplements without direction, well you can, but it will not be as effective. Find someone that really knows what they are doing and they can test you and your blood for certain things. (I recommend a "Live-Blood Analysis" if you can get one.) This can generate a realistic set of supplements you need to obtain. It is not just as simple as going to the health food store and asking the clerk "what should I take?" And with all due respect to our Allopathic doctors, most of them either do not know enough about high quality supplements or they do not think they are effective to treat medical imbalances. Supplements can make a HUGE difference in your health; but they can also be a near complete waste of your hard earned dollars if they are not the correct ones for your conditions.

BlogPost WEDNESDAY, MAY 03, 2006

## Still Walking

I got to do my presentation to the University of Arizona's Cancer Support Group on May 2nd. To say that I had butterflies in my stomach would be a mild understatement. Though I learned a long time ago if you have butterflies in your stomach the thing to do is **get them to fly in formation!**

The presentation went very well. I could not help but notice that the number of attendees was down by about one third to one half, but that is OK.

At the end of the presentation, during the question and answer period one of the social workers asked a really GREAT question.

**"What do you tell a patient that wants to do herbs, but his or her Oncologist refuses to let them?"**

The reason I like this question so much is it came from the audience, but it addresses *exactly* the issue at hand. Patients are requesting acupuncture for all kinds of issues and one of the road blocks they run into is: their Allopathic doctors.

What did I answer? Well, one of my challenges in life is I seem to be blunt. Honest, but direct. I said, "In my opinion what needs to happen is we need to open a dialogue with the oncologist, to allay any concerns he or she may have. **But, in the final analysis it is entirely up to the patient. The patient is the one that is experiencing the side effects of the chemotherapy, and it is THE PATIENTS BODY AND THE PATIENTS LIFE.** We just have to inform and support that patient as he or she makes his or her own decision."

The audience took that with mixed response. The ones that are truly patient advocates were ready to applaud. Others were not as enthused...

I am respectful of the doctors that are concerned about introducing herbs into the process of chemotherapy, but I want to address the concern head on, with factual information and research. I feel that many times what I am addressing is not factual concerns, but rather concerns born from lack of knowledge.

One very exciting part of the presentation was when one of the doctors said he wants to get acupuncture available in the new cancer hospital the University is building. That was great news...

But as I always say: "If you put that with $2 you can get a cup of coffee downtown. That is all it is worth." At this point in time.

Posted by Michael Clifford, L. Ac.

# Chapter 6

## Body Work ~ *Tui Na*

In ancient times it was common to study the martial arts with the healing arts. Out of this mix, Oriental Medicine has developed a very effective system of body work. The Chinese pronounce it as "Twee Na," in Japan it is called "*Shiatsu.*"

When a practitioner is well trained she/he can treat many, if not most conditions. *Tui Na* or *Shiatsu* is based on the same principles as Oriental medicine. The main difference is that the practitioner uses his body to affect the change in his patient as opposed to using needles or herbs. There are certain conditions that respond very well to effective *Tui Na* or *Shiatsu*.

Of course these two types of bodywork are very well suited for musculoskeletal conditions; but it would be inaccurate to think that is all they treat.

*Tui Na* is the first step in many treatments. If dealing with your thinking and diet has not cleared your condition or let you return to balance, it is time to get physical. With consistent *Tui Na* or *Shiatsu* treatments many conditions will balance themselves out. But you must be patient and willing to go through the full course of the treatments.

*Tui Na* or *Shiatsu* is not like regular bodywork. It penetrates deeply and a good practitioner brings you to and holds you on the edge of intensity necessary to get the job done. I do not mean to imply it is painful, it is intense at times, but it is also very relaxing. But when they let you get up you feel GREAT! Rejuvenated and refreshed for a nice change.

*Tui Na* and *Shiatsu* treatments incorporate pressing, stretching, deep compression of the muscles and gentle shaking of the limbs and joints. It is very good body work, usually done fully clothed and traditionally you would be on a tatami or futon mat.

BlogPost FRIDAY, APRIL 08, 2005

## More Subtle than Physical

I have been supervising a student clinic for the Asian Institute of Medical Studies; the clinic is a Tui Na Clinic in an Assisted Living Center. I have had two students last quarter and they returned for another quarter that will end at the end of May. It has been a great clinic.

One of the things that is always interesting to me is to see these patients respond so well from Tui Na. The bodywork has to be gentle, due to the age of the patients and their frail conditions. But almost always they respond very clearly to the bodywork. Old age has been called a second childhood and it is interesting to note that the seniors seem to respond to Tui Na as quickly as an infant does. Maybe it is because they are so close to the gate that their body responds to energy work more quickly than an adolescent or adult. Tui Na is well suited for this clientele; the gentle pressure is relaxing and relieves stagnation very effectively. Of course every patient is different, but with an average age of mid 80's we see a lot of stagnation and Qi deficiency.

One of the area's we have had to learn to work through is when a patient is non-verbal due to sequella of stroke. We have to become attuned to the individual patient and determine what works well for that patient on that day and adjust our treatments accordingly. Many times the students will start with a physical movement, a pressing or vibrating technique that will evolve naturally to the point their hand is not moving, but the vibration is 'internalizing' inside the musculature of the patient. As a supervisor I get to watch the patients from a different perspective than the students. I get to see the patient relax into this non-physical, vibrational form of treatment. It is cool to watch.

Posted by Michael Clifford, L. Ac.

## Acupuncture/Needle Work

So here we are, finally talking about acupuncture. You might have been wondering if we would ever get to this.

One of the most common questions I hear is "Does it hurt?" or some variation of that. So let's dive in there and then we can swim around a bit.

First of all, I will describe the needles themselves. An acupuncture needle is the diameter of 3-4 hairs, it is solid surgical stainless-steel and due to its size, it is flexible. There can be nothing inside a solid needle, so don't worry about that. The needles are what are called "Single use, sterile disposable needles." They get used on you, and <u>only</u> on you, and then they go into a biohazard disposal box and eventually get recycled.

When acupuncturists are going through their schooling, we are trained extensively on how to insert a needle without any pain. Yes, there are a few points that sting and or bite, but they are few. Really.

I remember treating one nice lady who was a little 'needle-phobic.' After the long intake process, I finally had her on the treatment table; I felt her pulses and looked at her tongue as described before. Then I started inserting the needles, I had about six of them in when she said "Now Michael, you know I am afraid of the needles so tell me before you stick me." I almost had to laugh as I told her, "I already have 6 needles in you. Every time you are exhaling on my command I have been inserting a needle." She said, "I have not felt anything!" This is actually not as rare or uncommon as you might think and it is not to say that I was a fantastic acupuncturist with skills far above and beyond mere mortals; though I might like you to think that occasionally.

When an acupuncturist is going to insert a needle he or she will press the plastic guide tube into your skin; this causes the nerves around it to sense and record that sensation. When the needle is inserted the tube is nearly simultaneously released and the nerves note that sensation. It is kind of a sleight-of-hand maneuver but essentially, we are tricking the nerves into not receiving one bit of information as they process another.

That is fine for needle insertion with guide tubes, but how did they do it before we had guide tubes? These are really new in acupuncture, having been used for less than 20 years. The acupuncturist would still guide your breathing and would either stretch your skin at the insertion site or would pinch it together depending on the location. Both ways change the elasticity of the skin and trick the nerves in a way that is similar to what we now accomplish with the guide tubes.

Either way the needle is inserted quickly to a depth below the surface layer of nerves; then it is guided to the specific depth required for that point on your body given your specific body type and size. By that, I mean that not everyone will have a needle inserted to the same depth for the same point as will another person with a different body type.

If I were to have to describe where and how *Qi* travels my current level of understanding leads me to consider the fascia (the sheath of connective tissue that surrounds the muscles and organs and is the largest tissue in the whole body, in fact it is an even larger organ than your skin) as the physical substrate that *Qi* <u>may</u> travel through. But since *Qi* is non-physical why would it require a physical substrate to travel in? This specific question is about why the fascia is NOT presumed to be the medium that *Qi* travels in, and yet there are many highly respected acupuncturists that believe the fascia is the medium in which *Qi* travels.

Propagation of symptoms during acupuncture treatments is "probably" the *Qi* traveling along meridians, but the nervous system does not explain the propagation of sensations. During testing it has been determined that *Qi* communication takes 12 times longer than nerve communication. It has also been determined that *Qi* does not travel along the same course as the nerve impulses are transmitted.

At times, I have encountered surgical complications, as when seeing a woman who had had surgery ten years previously for a hernia. She had been in constant pain since then. With only occasional relief, it has been an issue in her life since the day of the surgery.

She was told that it is due to the scars from the surgery and to have more surgery would probably only make things worse.

Ten years is a long time.

She came to me on the recommendation of a former patient and was basically at the point of "I have tried everything else; nothing else has helped. Maybe this will."

During the first treatment when I was palpating the site of the surgery I felt a scar about as big as my little finger, more or less. Same width and length. I did my regular type of treatment, but I also inserted needles directly into the ends of the scar.

When she came back in two weeks she was totally amazed to report that she had been nearly pain free for a week and a half. Not bad for one treatment...

The second treatment I branched out, quite a bit.

At the end of the treatment I worked on the scar with "invisible needles." At the lower end of her scar she said she could feel something like a thread being pulled out. Even I would have to say that is different.

After she got dressed and we were talking, she said something in her abdomen "released." The next time we talked, she had been nearly pain-free for the last two and a half weeks.

While that story involved invisible-needling, here's another experience involving physical needling that is somewhat mind-boggling.

I had the pleasure of treating a gentleman that had been surviving the effects of a stroke for nearly 30 years. When he was 29 years old he had a massive stroke as he was diving off a springboard into a pool. He did not discover acupuncture for nearly 28 years. He had been coming to the Acupuncture school nearly every week for the last two years and had been making steady progress. He was an interesting patient to deal with, and was always willing to try a new technique. I think I might have surprised him with my request.

The acupuncture school, The Asian Institute of Medical Studies, had a class for first-year students to observe a practitioner and see how she or he operated after graduation. I had done a few of these classes and it was a good experience for me; and from what I gather, it was good for the students as well. I got to meet new patients and the students got to watch as I 'did my thing.'

Enter this fine gentleman; He came into the room, with a cane and a smile. He had not been in "Observation Theatre" before, but as I said, he was a willing guy, so we were going through the questions. He slurred his words, but was able to communicate if you listened carefully.

Finally, I asked him to stick out his tongue. His tongue deviated sharply to the left; by that I mean that the last 1/4 of his tongue was turned at least 45 degrees to his left. And his tongue quivered while extended.

I talked to him about what I wanted to do. He listened to me and said, "You want to do WHAT?" I had explained to him that what I wanted to was to bleed the sublingual veins under his tongue. After we talked it over, he said "OK."

I bled the left vein then I needled the right vein with VERY STRONG STIMULATION. Actually, I stimulated the needle as strongly as he could stand. When I took the needle out of his tongue, he said CLEARLY "You'll never do that again!!!" Then he looked around for a minute and we could see this look of wonderment in his eyes as he realized that he was speaking clearly. I asked him to stick his tongue out again. It came out calmly and pointed straight forward.

Before leaving the clinic that day, he told us he was going to ask for that treatment again. He did, and his speech steadily improved.

Blogpost April 2006

I have been practicing a series of 'invisible needle' techniques. I have written a little about this before, but this is a slight variation. The theory of "5-element" or "5-Phase" acupuncture has a long history. There is an entire school of acupuncture that is based on this system. In short, it is an understanding that one "phase' of energy leads to, or creates, the next phase. I use the term phase because to my mind the concept of element implies static or unchanging; phase implies change. It is understood that these phases are dynamic.

This line of theory states that "Water creates Wood; Wood creates Fire; Fire creates Earth (the ashes of a fire a like earth/dirt); Earth creates Metal (in the earth there are veins of ore); Metal creates Water (near those veins of ore it is not uncommon to find underground rivers). That is the "creative" cycle. There is also a 'controlling' cycle. Water controls Fire (Water cools fire); Fire controls Metal (Fire melts Metal); Metal controls Wood (cuts); Wood controls Earth (the roots of a plant slowing erosion); Earth controls Water (Earthen dams, river banks). This is also seen as a family relationship; grandparents, parents and children. In an Asian family it is not uncommon to have three generations in one house and in that type of arrangement the grandparents have a lot of influence on the grandchildren.

What I have been working with is a variation of this where I am working to tonify one phase of energy, or more specifically one Organ system by treating it in a 5-phase context. Tonify the "mother" and sedate the "grandmother" to affect the energy of the "child." While that would be interesting to consider in terms of family dynamics, that is the subject for another book.

What is REALLY interesting is that in the clinic I supervise as well as with my own patients I am not physically touching the patient with the needle. Yet they are feeling the 'energy.' Here is what happens: At the end of a regular acupuncture treatment I feel the pulses once again, then depending on what their pulses are reflecting I perform an "invisible needle" treatment. I engage the patient by asking them to tell me when they feel the energy at the point. I hold the needle above the surface of their skin and work the needle the same as if it were "inserted." Every one of the patients has been reporting they feel this technique within 30 seconds. Way COOL!!!

Today I was working a point on the side of my patient's foot, but I still had the needles in the rest of her. I was stimulating a point on the Spleen meridian, Sp-2; she still had a needle in at Sp-3 (just across the knuckle of her big toe). Right before she said "I feel it" I watched the needle at Sp-3 make a huge movement; BUT I DID NOT SEE ANY MUSCULAR MOVEMENT IN ANY OF THE MUSCLES ON HER FOOT OR CALF. I finished the rest of her treatment and her pulses had changed considerably so it was time to let her go on with her day. But I am still thinking about that treatment.
As I said, this is SO weird!!!

Posted by Michael Clifford, L. Ac.

\*\*\*

When considering the intention of a specific acupuncture treatment here is what I try to contemplate.

Acupuncture is about "restoring balance" of the flow of *Qi* within one's body. Some situations manifest as a relative "excess" of energy within a particular meridian or *Organ System*, while others would manifest as a relative "deficiency" within a given meridian or *Organ System*. So this means that sometimes I would want to stimulate a point to allow the *Qi* to flow more evenly, and effortlessly. While other times I would want to stimulate the point in order for the *Qi* within that meridian to stimulate or build *Qi* within the related *Organ System*. That is what was meant by the previous statement of Rectify the *Qi*. Either way the entire process is <u>always</u> about restoring the balance of the free flow of *Qi* within the body.

## Auricular Treatments

There is another form of treatment that you may experience or have heard of: Ear Acupuncture; though in truth we do not have to use needles for this type of treatment.

Oriental Medicine has historical evidence of using the ears as a way to treat the body. Though the practice fell out of common use nearly a thousand years ago, it has been "rediscovered." The French have also advanced this form of treatment.

The theory is (whether it is Chinese or French, who cares?) that the body is completely represented in the ears (as well as the eyes, but that is another subject). When one is trained, he or she can visually inspect the ears for slight changes in coloration or texture and the area where changes are found will correspond to the area of the body that is out of balance. There are also new electronic devices that register a very slight change in electrical resistance between points and where that change in electrical resistance is where we find the slight change in coloration and or texture and the corresponding body system being out of balance.

All of the Organ Systems are represented as well as the joints (wrists, elbows, shoulders, complete spine, hips, knees and ankles), there are even points that correspond to endocrine glands (thyroid, hypothalamus, etc.). It is possible to treat the entire body by using only the ear, and you do not even have to use needles.

Just a quick word about needling the ears; these points are very commonly the most tender points to be found. Some people are very, very good at inserting a needle in and there is only a slight bite; other people are not as talented and it can hurt. But in a few seconds or a minute, that subsides and one is left with a warm relaxing sensation.

Auricular treatments are usually quite relaxing.

The U.S. Dept. of Justice has programs in some cities for treating non-violent substance-abuse cases that offer a convicted individual the choice of jail time or tightly guided probation with mandatory auricular treatments. They would not be doing this if there was no hard evidence that this can work. Auricular-detox treatments have a 30+ year history of clinical effectiveness in the U.S.

Blogpost MONDAY, MAY 08, 2006

## This is Truly Amazing

Every year I have to take a 'Continuing Education Course," the state, as well as the National Certification board requires at least 15 hours of training every year. I think this is a good thing and I have learned new things at every course I have taken. This year's was no exception, but it did raise the bar for others to compare with.

The course was called "Auricular Medicine." Dr.'s Huang and Huang, a husband and wife team from Taiwan have been researching auricular medicine for over 35 years. They have taken this medical art form into wholly new territory. After this week *I will never look at an ear in the same way.* Their way of looking and diagnosing is incredibly detailed, specific and backed by science.

When it came time to demonstrate they did NOT WANT ANY MEDICAL INFORMATION. They said, "We'll tell you and you can tell everyone here if it is correct." The first thing that caught my attention was when she looked at the volunteer's ear and said, "Oh, you snore at night." It was not a question. Visually she picked up several 'issues' that he confirmed. Then she started with the electrical detection machine. After several other issues she looks down to the floor and is quiet for a moment. Then she says, "You have hemorrhoids." Again not a question. She then looks at all of us watching and says "Sorry, no secrets here."

After the seminar while we were waiting for the plane I asked to have my ear checked over. My right hip has been sore for a few days. Either I am getting old or I just slept wrong a few day's earlier... ANYWAY, I had a seed put on the point the machine indicated. This morning my pain is about 90% gone!!!

My brother-in-law is a Judo guy. His knee was hurting, so after this seminar I asked if I could test him with this electrical device. He said "Sure, why not?" I found that the point for his right knee activated, whereas no other point on either ear did. I taped an "ear-seed" on to the point and forgot about it. I called him two days later to ask if there were any changes. He said his knee stopped hurting that evening and had not hurt him since. The ear-seed stayed in place for a week and he was pain-free for nearly 3 weeks. Go figure.

I am going to continue to check this out. To say I am curious would be an understatement.

Posted by Michael Clifford, L. Ac.

Earlier, I wrote about using 'auricular medicine' or ear seeds to treat some of the patients I serve. It has been interesting, sometimes these seeds work extremely well, and sometimes they do not seem to have a direct effect. I suspect that when there are not obvious results one or the other of two things has happened. Either I mis-located the seed (imagine close to 200 points on each ear, if you are off by "just a little bit" it is like you are choosing another point entirely), or the results are more subtle than we are seeing. That was not the case recently. I am treating a 52 y.o. woman for the complications from uterine fibroids. Her fibroids are approximately the size of a four-month-old fetus. She is going to have a complete hysterectomy and I do think that is a good choice considering how the fibroids are growing so rapidly. In the last six months they have grown from the size of few peas to their current dimensions. When one has a growth of that size it has to be addressed, and surgery might be the best choice. Anyway, from a TCM perspective, fibroids are one manifestation of blood stasis. The treatment then is to "Invigorate the Blood and Resolve the Stasis." Because she was scheduled for surgery I did not giving her herbs at this time. I used acupuncture and the ear seeds. Even though she was 52, she was still having a regular menstrual cycle. Two days later her period started; it was EXTREMELY HEAVY, to the point she was concerned about it. After four days of that she felt that the change/cause of this was the ear seeds. She removed them and within four hours her period had stopped. The point that I had the seed on was the 'uterus point.' I believe that the seed had activated the energy affecting her uterus and was "Invigorating the Blood." On a physical level, she felt better than she had in several months. I saw her after her surgery to restore the flow of the meridians that were disrupted by the surgery. What amazed me about this was how her cycle had changed so drastically and when she removed the seeds her period stopped in a few hours. I know that the ears are very effective but this was one of the most graphic examples I have seen.

# Chapter 7

## Herbal Treatments

There is some debate about where to place herbology in the continuum of invasive treatments. One argument is that one does not have to pierce, massage or manipulate the body; therefore it must be less invasive (in which case it would be earlier on my list). There is another argument that says even if I try really hard it is difficult to do serious damage to someone with acupuncture.

Yes, I could puncture a lung, but if you ever get to look at a cadaver you would see that I would actually have to either be totally ignorant of anatomy (in which case I should not be sticking needles into you) or it would have to be intentional or a very bizarre accident. But when it comes to herbology one can make choices that have serious consequences.

Make no mistake about it: ANY HERBAL MEDICINE CAN BE VERY POWERFUL, AND IT CAN HAVE SERIOUS ADVERSE EFFECTS ON YOUR HEALTH.

At the same time, there are conditions that many Oriental Medicine practitioners feel can only be treated effectively by taking herbal medicine.

It is a matter of being sure that your practitioner knows what he or she is doing. By way of explanation let me bounce back to the first over-simplified pattern of dis-harmony I talked about.

"John is 32 years old. Last night he was tired after work, and after dinner he took a shower and went to bed. This morning when he awakened he had a sore throat, and was feeling aches in his muscles. His wife felt his forehead and said he did not have a fever. That night when John came home he was very achy, he had a headache and he definitely had a fever."

If the practitioner does not pick up on some vital information in this very simplified pattern he or she can make a big mistake. On the first evening, John did not have a fever, but he did have one by the second evening. Let us say, for example, that the practitioner did not see the heat signs presenting in the second evening. Rest assured this is highly unlikely as this is one of the primary things we are trained to look for. The practitioner would then see a pattern of *wind-cold*, and follow the dictum "If there is Cold, Warm it". That would mean that he or she would very possibly add "warming herbs" to any formula being created.

If one already has heat and then one adds warming herbs to that you can rapidly get a very bad response. This is my main concern with just going to a health food store that also sells Chinese herbs and asking the store clerk which formula to take. "Oh, my sister had a cold last month, this worked great for her". I don't know about you, but I have not had good luck trying to put a fire out by adding fuel to it. And I have never found "one-size fits all" to be applicable in matters of health.

No disrespect to the store clerk intended. I actually worked as a store clerk in a health food store just after graduating and I had to bite my tongue when people would ask me for this type of advice. I usually responded with a guarded answer to direct them to either see me professionally or seek other professional medical advice if needed.

There are conditions or patterns of dis-harmony, however, that will only respond well to herbs. These are almost always patterns that have been developing for quite a while, and they are also almost always patterns of a more 'internal nature.' I am thinking of *Blood* disorders, digestive disorders as well as Western blood disorders.

One reason I think these patterns require herbs is because they have penetrated our beingness so deeply. It is like the needles can't quite get there.

One of the best reasons to properly use herbs would be their nearly infinite ability to be uniquely and specifically tailored for each individual at every stage of their recovery. When someone makes a traditional herbal formula they are drawing on thousands of years of empirical experience. Some formulas I used have a documented history of over 2,000 years. I could use that formula as it was written, or I could modify it because it is comprised of measured loose herbs. I could add to or subtract herbs from the base formula to create a formula for your unique condition.

Another great point for herbal formulas is how they are 'balanced', by this I mean to acknowledge that everything we put into our body has effects and "side-effects." A good formula will achieve a balance of building or tonifying with 'moving' or 'dispersing'; it will balance warming with cooling so that the overall effect is the desired effect. And these herbs have been studied for thousands of years, on millions of people of all different states of health, gender and age ranges. In other words, if someone is well trained in herbology, they have a lot of information at their disposal; even more than an acupuncturist; very possibly more than a Western doctor.

By balancing a formula in the intricate ways that herbology allows, one can create gentle yet effective formulas. That is not to say the tea will taste good. The process one has to work through at home of soaking then boiling, draining, refilling and boiling again combined with the aroma of the herbs in your house is enough to make many of us say "Forget about it!" But if you make it that far, depending on the condition you are treating the taste may be from sweet to very bitter. It all depends.

I remember my first experience with a loose herb formula. It is not one I will soon forget. I was living in Seattle at the time, running my martial-arts school and teaching full-force Women's Self-Defense courses. It was a great time in my life! But I developed a whole body rash with bright-red dots appearing everywhere. (I did not know it at the time, but this was a reaction to extended exposure to a heating balm I had been putting on my knees.) There was an acupuncture school just around the corner from my school. I went in for treatments; their diagnosis was Heat, almost at *Blood* level. (That would be BAD.) After the treatment, they gave me a written formula for the loose herbs I was to take. I went down to the International District to get the formula filled. When I got home and followed the steps to make this concoction my apartment had odors I had never experienced before. Then I poured a cup of this tea and sat out in front to read and drink my 'tea'. First sip, I nearly gagged! Oh My God! I am supposed to drink this twice a day?? The funny thing was, by the end of the second cup I was okay with the taste and by the end of the second day, I actually liked it. What was going on here?

When a formula is correct for your condition your body will respond to it in a myriad of ways. One way is that the taste will become more palatable; another way is that the condition you are treating will start to subside. My rash was gone before my next week's acupuncture appointment.

If you are unable, or unwilling to make the raw herb tea there are capsules and tablets one can take in place of drinking the tea. The primary advantage of capsules or tablets is that patients will probably have a better compliance rate than those brewing and drinking teas. The other side of this is that the formula is predetermined and while it is probably a good formula, it cannot be modified. Also the differences between one manufacturer and another can be fairly significant. This is why I would use one supplier for some patients but for another patient with a similar but not identical pattern I would use a different supplier. Some versions of a formula are more 'warming' or 'cooler' than others; some are more 'moving' some are less moving. So the practitioner has to be aware of these differences in each manufacturer's formulas.

I would talk to my patient's to see what they thought and felt about the herbs. For a very few patients I would very strongly urge them to make the tea and drink it because where they were in their healing process was going to be better served by the infinite flexibility of loose herb formulas. When they improved we could go to capsules and or tablets.

Also, when I was supervising in the student clinic at the Asian Institute of Medical Studies we had a patient that had a serious, life-threatening condition. Her blood did not clot; she had a genetic condition that will always be with her. Can you imagine, for a paper cut she will HAVE to go to the hospital, it is not a choice; her blood will continue to seep and or spurt out until she gets Western medicine to stop it. She said she has to put a towel over her hand, hold it with tight compression and go immediately to the emergency room. That would be for a very minor cut, for a serious cut it would be much more serious. For this reason she is on continual birth-control, which I actually support and agree with. When she was leaving I talked to her about an idea I had for her. There is a herbal powder available in most Chinese herbal stores called "*Yunan Bai Yao*" that we use to stop bleeding. In fact, during the war in Vietnam many times our soldiers would find a bottle of it, with its 'red emergency pill' in the pockets of dead Vietnamese soldiers. But they did not know why. I told this woman to go buy some and keep it with her, in her purse or somewhere where it will ALWAYS be accessible. The next time she gets cut, she was to sprinkle some on the cut AND go to the hospital. I got a report after she suffered another cut. She was freaking out, as you can imagine. Then she remembered the *Yunan Bai Yao*. She sprinkled it in and on the cut. She told her intern that she could literally see the blood stop flowing. She was able to just put a band aid over the cut and was fine. Now of course I am gonna tell you "Don't try this at home!" But in all honesty, I think it could be of great value, and especially if you live in a remote area. It is amazing stuff, and it works.

BlogPost SUNDAY, DECEMBER 24, 2006

## Ginger, as you have never thought about it before

A few weeks ago my Mom was telling me about an article she read; I believe it was in Newsweek. Anyway it was "Health from A-Z." I was expecting her to mention acupuncture, or Chinese Herbal medicine. She surprised me, as she is known for doing.

N is for nutrient. The one that she was telling me about is Ginger, or what we call Sheng Jiang. Settles the stomach, warms the center. Is also gaining recognition for its effectiveness in helping stop chemotherapy induced nausea. That was all well and good, but not surprising.

What surprised me was when she told me it is being tested for treating ovarian cancer. I was very surprised to learn that it is effective in killing ovarian cancer cells.

I had to read up on that. Here is a quote from the article linked mentioned above, "In laboratory studies, researchers found ginger caused ovarian cancer cells to die. Further, the way in which the cells died suggests ginger may avoid the problem common in ovarian cancer of cells becoming resistant to standard treatments."

Let's take a second to think this through. Then I will go off on my tangent... as usual.

If one could use a natural herbal product to kill cancer, why are we not hearing about this? Well to be sure, it has to be investigated more thoroughly. That is obvious and essential.

The type of ginger they use is a powdered form, not the sheng jiang form, but the "Gan Jiang" form. In TCM's perspective it is spicy and hot. It "Warms the Spleen and Stomach and dispels Cold." It also dispels Internal Cold.

TCM has many different ways of looking at and conceptualizing cancer. Two that resonates with me are "Lingering Pathogens, and Latent Heat" but what is interesting here is that I would see this as using Fire to fight Fire. As a former fire-fighter I can see the validity of that approach. If you can burn out the fuel before it spreads you can actually contain the fire.

Of course always remember that when I use the term "fire" in this context I do not mean the same as what is burning the logs in your fireplace. In the same way as when I mention organs "I do not mean the bio-medical physical-substrate organ. I mean the energy that "runs" the organ. Or in this example the energetics of this dis-ease that manifest as, or have the function of fire. "It is the same thing, only completely different."

So back to the article: "If ginger causes the cancer cells to die and in such a way that they may not become resistant to other treatments it could hold a huge potential."

What I am wondering is: is there a way that this could be applied directly. Through laparoscopy could a GYN surgeon directly apply ginger as a paste to the cancerous cells on a woman's ovaries? I know about liability, but look at it this way, if a woman is being faced with death, or chemotherapy that will honestly make her wish she was dead at times; would it not make sense to try this. There are organic farmers, get the ginger, dry it out while the lawyers are finessing release of liability forms, then apply it directly to the cells.

What can happen? Well if it is as hot as TCM sees it she may be uncomfortable, that is true and maybe it will be too hot, maybe not. They can flush it out if it is too hot. If not, well maybe it will stop the cancer. Maybe it will not. But if it does not she still has the same choices as before.

BUT WHAT IF IT DOES WORK?

Think about that. I do not know the statistics right off, but I do know that ovarian cancer is a deadly serious condition. Don't we owe it to all the women in our lives to try something like this? If it does not work, there would be no damage done. TCM has used ginger for thousands of years, internally and externally.

The statistics are easy, the same article says: "More than 20,000 women are expected to be diagnosed with ovarian cancer this year, and 15,000 will die from the disease, according to the American Cancer Society. "

For information about ovarian cancer, go to www.cancer.med.umich.edu/learn/ovarianinfo.htm or call the U-M Cancer Answer Line at 800-865-1125."

I think this needs to be explored, and not discarded unless it proves that it does not work. But the study from the University of Michigan seems to have promise

http://www.med.umich.edu/opm/newspage/2006/ginger.htm

Posted by Michael Clifford, L. Ac.

## Duration of Treatments

In general, there are two simple ways to look at how long you will have to get treatments. First of all, if it is a sudden onset, like a pulled muscle, or a "cold" your body will probably respond well and in one or two treatments you will be noticing big results; in fact, the condition may even be resolved. But if the condition is one you have been dealing with for a while it will take some time to resolve the underlying cause of the effect you are experiencing.

We usually expect a longer term condition to take "one month of treatment for every year you have had it." This can be quite disheartening, I know. But what I want you to consider is that you did not get into the state of imbalance you are currently in overnight, and it is unrealistic to expect to resolve it overnight as well.

Acupuncture and Oriental Medicine are subtle medicines. They do work in very powerful ways; but they also work slowly while adjusting many of the underlying causes of the imbalance we are experiencing.

Western medicine treats the symptoms; OM treats the "root cause". One works faster, but does not truly address the *cause* in many cases; the other works slower but deeper. There is a time and a place for each system.

Even when you are in optimal health, it is wise and recommended to get five treatments a year, one for every change of season. And you thought there were only four seasons.

BlogPost SATURDAY, APRIL 22, 2006

## Surrounding the Dragon

This week I had the pleasure of meeting and treating a lady that has had severe, chronic neck pain for the last 17 years. It causes severe headaches, almost daily.

Whenever I do an intake I always ask about pain. I ask my patient to 'quantify' the pain on a one-to-ten scale, with ten being unbearable. Once I had a young woman say her headaches were about a 13. OUCH!!! was all I could say. This week's lady said her pain was about 9 and her headache so far (10:30 a.m.) was only a 4. I think she would have went for higher numbers, but wanted to work within the scale presented to her...

As I was palpating the muscles on and around her shoulder blade I felt a knot, about the size of my thumb. The whole thumb. I decided it was time to "Surround the Dragon."

One of the techniques we use for a situation like this is to insert needles around the knot and let the needles start to break-up the stagnation that is manifesting as a knot. When I put the needles into her back she felt an "unwinding" sensation in the area.

After 15 minutes or so I removed the needles and did a Tui-Na release treatment on her neck and shoulders. The muscles on the top of her shoulders are tighter than a towing cable. It was like pushing into a table top. Unbelievable tension. No wonder she gets headaches.

I decided to stretch the envelope a little more. I inserted an 'intra-dermal' needle into the tightest part of the top of her shoulder, taped it over, talked it over and sent her home.

Here is the nutshell of what I said: "The intra-dermal needle is extremely small, but by leaving it in place it will continue to release the tension in your shoulder muscles and should help with your headaches. If it gets to be too much remove the tape, it is taped in place in such a way that removing the tape will pull the needle out. But be sure to look and see the needle in the tape. If it does not come out someone else will have to search it out and use tweezers to remove it."

That actually is a fairly common treatment, it is just unusual for me to do that on the first visit. But she was in such pain that I felt compelled to extend the treatment if possible.

When she left she was feeling so much better, the pain was down to a 4 and her headache was gone.

It's a good start.

Posted by Michael Clifford, L. Ac.

BlogPost TUESDAY, APRIL 25, 2006

## Chipping Away

This week I got to see the lady with the neck pain.

Her pain level has dropped from the 9 level it was to a consistent 5.

That is huge, and I do appreciate this change. But not as much as my patient does. ;-)

She said "I am almost afraid to talk about it because I do not want to jinx whatever you've done."

The trapezius muscle at the top of her shoulder has loosened up so it is now more like a rope instead of a steel cable. It is progress, to be sure. But it's not over, this I know.

The morning I saw her she had had a migraine, that had to have pain relief, medication style. When I saw her the headache had dropped to a 2. When she left she was happy, relaxed and pain-free. I will keep chipping away at this. I know it will be resolved, and that she is in a much better position than she has been for the last 17 years...

Posted by Michael Clifford, L. Ac.

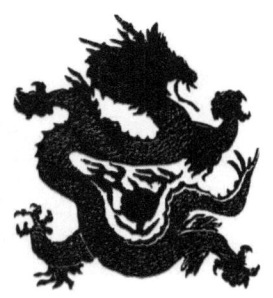

# Part Three

# Chapter 8

When discovering and describing the concepts of Oriental Medicine the Ancients also observed nature. Their detailed patient observations led them to recognize patterns, and then patterns within the patterns.

Oriental Medicine is strongly based upon relationships. We all need to understand our relationships with nature and the effects of that on our health. It was observed that things in nature tend to happen in cyclic patterns and the Ancients observed the same within our own bodies. As we have all observed, each season builds, crests, and then recedes as the next season starts to build; it is the same within our lifetimes as well.

The issue of relationships is interesting to contemplate, but first let me describe the idea behind the term "Elements." It is relatively agreed upon in academic circles now that the term 'element' is an inaccurate translation. More accurately it would be "phase." Our understanding of 'element' commonly causes one to think of 'unchanging' and that is exactly the <u>opposite</u> of what this concept entails.

In Oriental Medicine, it seems as though nothing is static and unchanging. This is true in nature as well as in our bodies and health.

In describing the phases as I am going to do, it will be important for you to let go of some of the preconceived ideas we all have about the terms I use. As I said earlier, the same word can have many different meanings. I am going to use familiar words, but in an unfamiliar context and meaning.

# Cycles

It has been observed that there are three primary cycles we can observe; generation, control and "insulting" (or reverse-control). These terms will be explained in more detail, but essentially they are what they appear to mean.

One reason I do not get too specific on these definitions is that I want you to be required to use your own imagination and not my limitations, but I also want to steer you in the general direction.

**GENERATION:** *this is the cycle of building, or creating. Each of the phases has a name from the natural environment and that will help us understand their co-relations.*

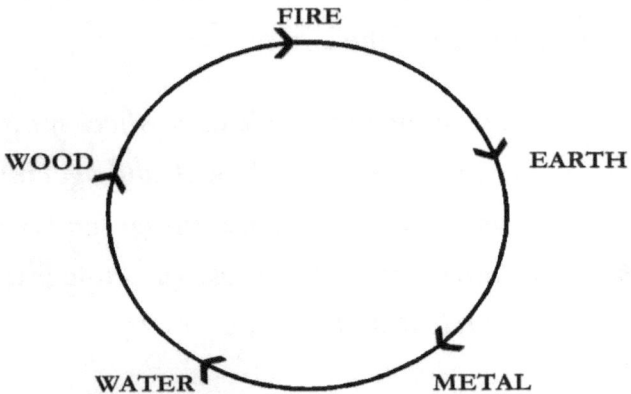

Wood represents expansion, or outward movement in all directions; wood can bend and be straightened. *Wood generates Fire*

Fire is said to "Flare upwards" and represents upward movement. *Fire generates Earth* (Ashes are earth-like).

Earth represents stability, sowing, growing and reaping; Earth also represents neutrality. *Earth generates Metal.* (In the earth are veins of ore.)

Metal represents contractive inward movement; and Metal can be molded and can harden. *Metal Generates Water* (Near the veins of ore one commonly finds underground rivers or water; and when metal is left out overnight water will condense on it.)

Water represents downward movement and moistens. *Water generates Wood*

The cycle repeats and the continual generation of each phase continues. This is commonly depicted in a circle with five points, each representing one phase going 'clockwise' with Fire traditionally placed at the top of the circle.

*{CONTROL: if you visualize the cycle as a wheel spinning and adding speed, it would be easy to see how it could get out of control. Therefore, it has been observed that things tend to intersect or exert a form of control on other things. The same is true within the five phases of Oriental Medicine.*

**Wood controls Earth**. I think of the roots of trees or grass penetrating into the earth preventing erosion.

***Earth controls Water.*** Here I think of river banks or earthen dams holding back the waters.

***Water controls Fire.*** Think of the cooling action of water being sprayed on a fire.

***Fire controls Metal.*** Fire can melt metal; if that is not control I do not know what is!

***Metal controls Wood.*** A metal axe is used to cut wood.

This cycle is usually represented as a five-pointed star, again with Fire at the top point of the star.

These two cycles are the most common and can be fairly easily understood. In my practice I almost always introduced this concept in my initial intake and treatment and it usually takes less than 5 minutes to cover.

Together these two cycles look like this:

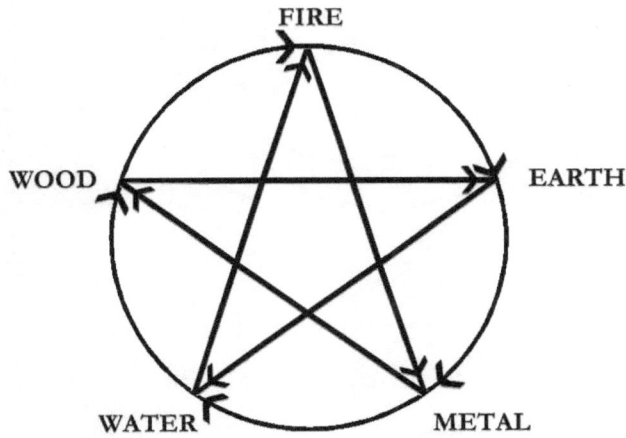

The next cycle is the reverse of the control cycle, it is commonly called the "INSULTING CYCLE," here is how I talked about it: "In traditional Asian families it is common to have three generations living within the same house. This is becoming more common in our society as well. In a situation like this, the Grandparents have a lot of influence on the Grandchildren as the Parents are 'out in the field earning a living.' It is normal and accepted that the grandparents will be guiding and teaching the grandchildren, correcting them as needed and teaching them as they can. It is considered to be an insult if the grandchildren *talk back* to the grandparents. I wish this was more clearly understood within our society."

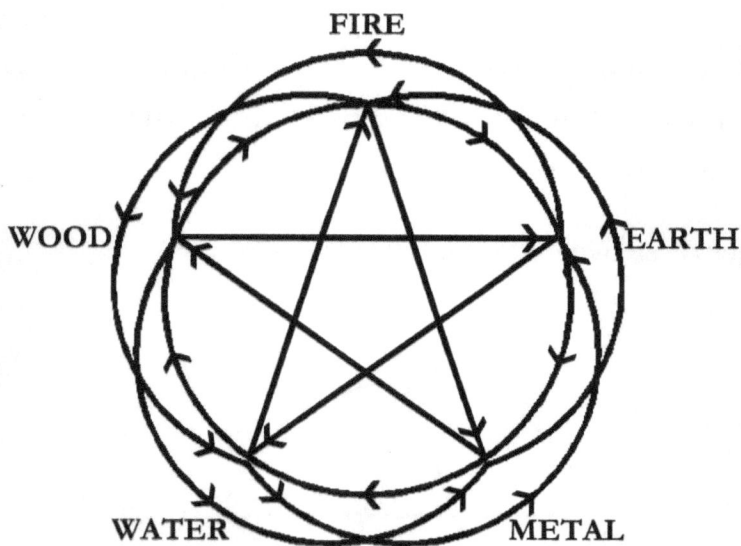

The Insulting cycle can be understood more clearly when I explain about the inter-relationship of emotions and health. The insulting cycle can be visualized as either a 5 pointed star, with the arrows "in the opposite direction," or as I depict above as a series of arcs connecting one phase to another, but traveling in the opposite direction of all the other flows.

There are entire schools of Oriental Medicine that are entirely devoted to the five-phase system. They are very good schools and they turn out very good acupuncturists. I do find the five-phase system to be quite useful; the inter-relationship of the phases and their corresponding Organ Systems makes it easier to explain to the general public.

As a slight digression I just want to remind you that there are multiple ways of understanding Oriental Medicine, and that each one may be self-reliant but it does fit in with every other system of Oriental Medicine. It is not like I have to abandon one set of theories to grapple with another; they all fit together and the strengths of one system compensate for the weaknesses of another system. And every system, whether Western or Eastern has its unique strengths and its own peculiar weaknesses.

## Freezing Wind

I remember one incredibly complex scenario to describe how one can have "Wind" and yet be "frozen" in the extreme. Here is what I mean: The doctor told her she had a tumor in her brain and that surgery was the best option. When they got into the tumor they found that it had grown around an artery in her brain. While scraping the tumor off the artery, the artery was 'nicked' and she had a massive stroke. She survived, but will never be the same. The right side of her face is severely affected, her speech is seriously impaired, as well as her walking and all right-side body movements.

That was two years ago. Countless hours of rehab later she is still only able to walk with a walker or a cane. Most times out of the house she will be in her chair, as it is easier overall.

I had the pleasure of meeting and treating this beautiful soul. We have been working together on a weekly basis for 4 weeks now. Her face is still paralyzed, but she is starting to get some tingling sensations around her eye and in her cheek.

This beautiful soul is teaching me about perseverance, and perspective.

Those of you that know me can imagine how I would respond to this if it were me. I am not even sure the doc could have convinced me to let them open up my skull and perform the surgery. Much less what my reaction would have been to the aftermath of that surgery...

This beautiful woman has realized that there is some reason she is still alive. She may not be happy, but she is not unhappy. She may long to do some things but she can accept that she cannot do everything as she used to do. Through all of our time together she is so positive, yet realistic. It humbles me.

From a TCM perspective we talk about a stroke as "internal wind" because it strike so fast like wind and it is internally generated. The shaking of Parkinson's disease, the twitching of a facial muscle, a gran-mal seizure; all of these are manifestations of Internal Wind.

I added the term "frozen" on because the sequela of a stroke leaves the face muscles "frozen" in place. Bell's palsy is a very good example, and it is one that responds well to acupuncture and herbs. (In fact if you ever have Bell's palsy, or know someone that does, send them to an acupuncturist ASAP!)

The treatment for Internal Wind is to nourish the Liver, Extinguish the Wind, and to Calm the Shen (spirit). We are proceeding with this, but because of the medications she is on I will not risk using herbs. Chinese herbology can be very effective in treating stroke, but I will not risk that for her, at this time. Maybe later...

But for me, for today I am just feeling humbled by this beautiful, powerful soul. It really does help put my life into perspective....

# Chapter 9

# Organ Systems

In this section I am going to give out a lot of information. You may want to read about one organ system that intrigues you first or come back to this as a reference. I feel the degree of information I am imparting is fairly significant, and I want it to be available if it is of interest to you. I am trying to find the appropriate balance.

When I speak of Organ Systems, it is important to remember that I am not referring to any Western Biomedical understanding of any organ. There are similarities, to be sure; but there are also worlds of difference. Please keep that in mind.

Imagine my hands in front of my body at about shoulder height with my elbows bent so that the palms are facing out. My hands can easily describe circles in their relaxed movement. These circles could be seen to represent each system of medicine's understanding of an organ's function. There will be an area in the middle where the two overlap, but there will be a larger area where each one is separate. In some cases as I describe the Organ Systems it will be like my hands are as far apart as I can reach, with no overlapping area. For some there will be a larger degree of overlap.

For each Organ System I will describe its primary function, the emotion that is expressed through it, the color and taste associated with it, and its place in the five-phase theory. I will also pair it with its corresponding partner. (Note: the "*Yang* Organs" do not have emotions associated with them.)

# Lungs/Large Intestines

### LUNGS     Yin Organ

The Lungs primary function is to govern *Qi* and respiration; to control the meridians and Blood vessels; to regulate the Water passages, and to control the skin and hair. It is said the Lungs "open into the nose."

- The primary function of the Lungs is to govern $Qi$ and respiration. This means that they work to gather the clean and pure $Qi$ from the air and bring it into our bodies so we can utilize the $Qi$ of the air.

- Regulating the Water passages is about making sure the other Organ Systems have an adequate supply of moisture.

- Controlling the skin and hair is about regulating whether or not the pores of our skin open to allow us to sweat at the appropriate times as well as keeping our pores closed to prevent us from sweating at incorrect times.

By the Lungs 'opening to the nose' is recognition of the obvious that we breathe through our noses, but also that when an external pathogen does invade our body its primary opportunity will be through breathing through our nose.

It is said that the emotion of the Lungs is 'grief.' This makes sense when I think of the heavy sobbing of losing a loved one. It is also common that when someone has experienced a lot of grief in their life he or she will have weak Lung $Qi$. It is also common for a person that has some type of lung dysfunction (emphysema or asthma) to have a greater degree of grief in their life.

In five-phase theory the Lungs are associated with Metal, their color is white, their 'flavor' (that they respond to) is pungent, or aromatic, and the season is autumn.

In five-phase theory, Metal controls Wood, so this means the Lungs control the Liver. What this *could* mean is if someone's Lung *Qi* is deficient there would not be enough control/restraint on the Liver which *could* allow the Liver Yang to rise possibly manifesting as a headache at the very top of your head or for the Liver *Qi* to *stagnate* which may manifest as anger or irritability. Or as I have observed in various patients, first you get sad, and then you get a headache or get angry. In an "insulting Cycle" of the five phase theory the Lung *Qi* would 'insult' or travel back to the Heart; possibly manifesting as being easily startled, or developing insomnia or forgetfulness.

Lung dis-harmonies may manifest as:

- *Qi* Deficiency: This is where you feel tired, lethargic all the time for no apparent reason.

- Stagnant Lung *Qi:* Where you have a cough, which may or may not include dryness -- manifesting as a dry cough, or a dry scratchy throat.

- Yin Deficiency :Dryness in the nose and throat and mild heat signs.

- Accumulation of "Dampness": Here the Spleen is not transforming fluids, causing the Lungs to have problems associated with liquefying and disseminating the fluids.

- Heat in Lungs: Lung Fire, which manifest as yellow-green mucous, and/or may lead to constipation.

# LARGE INTESTINE     Yang Organ

The primary function of the Large Intestine is to receive food and drink from the Small Intestine. Having re-absorbed some of the fluids, it excretes the stools.

**Relationship to the Lungs**

The Lungs and Large Intestine are related to one-another, and both are on the interior, yet connected to the exterior. This relationship is important for the execution of common bodily functions, such as when descending Lung *Qi* lends the Large Intestine the necessary *Qi* for the effort of defecation.

If the Lung *Qi* is deficient, it does not give enough *Qi* to the Large Intestine for the act of defecation, resulting in constipation. This is particularly common with older people with deficient Lung *Qi*.

Conversely, the Lungs ability to send *Qi* downwards depends on the Large Intestine's role in excreting waste food material. If this function is impaired and there is constipation, the stagnation of food in the Large Intestine may impair the Lungs descending function giving rise to breathlessness.

Because the Large Intestine is related to the Lungs (as stated before, both are interior and yet are connected to the exterior), all of the five-phase associations are the same.

Duties of the Large Intestine: works as, and sometimes is known as, 'the garbage picker.'

- The Large Intestine governs body fluids; this is part of its function of reabsorbing fluids as it receives the waste from Small Intestine for elimination.

Looking at how the Lungs and Large Intestines are in Relationship we see that the Lungs circulate and descend *Qi*. However Lung heat can dry out stools which can cause Large Intestine Stagnation constipation and that could cause Dyspnea (difficult breathing)

One thing you may find if you receive acupuncture treatments is that because of their "interior/exterior" relationship the Large Intestine Meridian is frequently used to disperse Lung Heat.

Most Large Intestine disorders can be explained and treated by Spleen dis-harmonies. Acupuncture schools do not teach Large Intestine disorders and we will look at those disorders while considering the Spleen.

## Stomach/Spleen

### STOMACH      Yang Organ

The primary function of the Stomach is to "rot and ripen" the food before it sends the coarse *Qi* to the Spleen for transformation. The Stomach is one of the most Important Yang Organs, because without a healthy Stomach there would be inadequate nourishment.

The Stomach is associated with the Earth Phase; the color is Yellow, and the flavor is sweet. The Earth Phase does not have a season associated with it; though at the end of each season it is said to be in the Earth Phase as it transforms from one season to the next.

In five phase theory Earth controls Water, and the "Insulting Cycle" would be Earth insulting Metal, or the Stomach/Spleen insulting the Liver/Gallbladder. Trust me, the Stomach is almost never strong enough to attack the Liver, but the opposite will frequently happen as we will discuss.

The Stomach is the 'source and root' of all fluids because it is the repository where all fluids enter the body. This means that the Stomach is the source of all Yin (Remember Yin is substantive). Because the Stomach is the root and source of all Yin that means that the Stomach dislikes dryness and heat, as they tend to dry out Yin.

The Duties of the Stomach: To receive and decompose food (or as the Ancient's would say to 'rot and ripen'), and transmit nutrients to the limbs.

- Stomach dis-harmonies may manifest as: the common pain or stomach ache, distension (where your stomach is bloated), nausea, vomiting, and or belching (but this can come from invasion by Liver, which would be distinguished by other signs).

If there is excess heat or dryness in your body, and particularly your Stomach you may develop Stomach Yin deficiency manifesting as Excess Heat or "Stomach Fire" where there is a 'burning sensation' in your stomach with a high thirst for COLD liquids.

The Spleen & Stomach in Relationship: This is a very close relationship, often referred to as the stomachspleen. As a prime example, look at these concepts – the Spleen rules ascending *Qi*, whereas the Stomach rules descending *Qi*. Can you see how these two are intertwined and have to be in balance? This means that dis-harmonies of one often affect the other.

## SPLEEN     Yin Organ

The primary function of the Spleen is to *transform Qi*. It is the Spleen that changes the food energy we consume into energy our body can use. In my opinion the Spleen is one of the most important Organ Systems in our body.

I remember when I was in the Student Clinic at *Southwest Acupuncture College* during my first trimester of actually doing the treatments (which was in my second year). I was treating a nice elder. I think he was about 75. When I was feeling his pulses I commented that his Spleen pulse was deep and weak. He said "Yeah, they cut that out 25 years ago. I imagine it would be weak by now." Once I quit laughing I explained that the concept of the Spleen in Oriental Medicine is not the same as the spleen in Western Medicine.

This is a really good example of the different paradigms of medicine. In Western Medicine it is understood that the spleen has some immunological function, but they are still not sure what exactly its full role is; other than that it is sometimes thought of as an evolutionary-holdover. If the spleen gets injured or infected the primary choice of action would be to remove it, in an operation called a splenectomy. But even if the spleen was removed 25 years ago, there is still a Spleen Pulse; because if the Spleen is not able to *transform* the *Qi* your body will die.

In Oriental Medicine, the Spleen is of primary importance. The Spleen's duties of "Transforming and Transporting" the *Qi* is paramount to good health. One of my teachers even used to say "When you run into a truly complicated case, if you cannot find a clear thread to follow, start by tonifying the Spleen and the Kidneys. You will unravel a lot of the complications that way." He is correct.

As with the Stomach, the Spleen is associated with the Earth Phase; the color is Yellow, and the flavor is sweet. The emotion of the Spleen is "Pensiveness" I like this definition: *quiet modes of apparent or real thought.*

In Five-Phase Theory, the Earth Phase controls the Water Phase, or the Spleen/Stomach controls the Kidneys/Urinary Bladder. The Earth Phase is controlled by the Wood Phase, or the Liver/Gallbladder controls the Spleen/Stomach. It is rare for the "Insulting Cycle" to happen from the Earth insulting the Wood. The Liver is usually too darn strong and in a bad mood anyway.

- The Spleen is also known as "The Official in Charge of Transportation and Transformation". The Spleen *transforms* fluids to mists, food to *Qi*, and *transforms thoughts.* (There's one to keep you wondering !)

- The Spleen opens to the mouth, and distinguishes the five flavors. The Spleen is able to transport the flavors to where they need to go (which is important in herbal prescriptions). If Spleen *Qi* is notably deficient, one must tonify the Spleen before implementing other treatments, especially herbal remedies because if the Spleen cannot transform the *Qi* of the herbs it will only cause the person to become bloated.

- The Spleen manifests in the lips, the lips are a 'window' into the vitality of the Spleen, if the Spleen *Qi* is deficient the lips will be pale.

- The Spleen dislikes Dampness & Cold. Or as my teacher said, "Ice Cream puts out the spleen fire." Also consider that the Stomach dislikes Heat and Dryness, so we have a dynamic tension that has to be balanced. The Spleen dislikes Cold and the Stomach dislikes Heat, yet we all ingest both Cold and Heat frequently.

- The Spleen helps to hold blood into place, in the vessels, in the uterus, literally everywhere. The Spleen is also responsible for *Up-bearing*, which means it literally holds organs up. The Spleen also is integral to *Raising*, which means it sends food *Qi* to Lungs where it starts the process of making Blood.

- Most importantly, the Spleen has the property of Transforming. It transforms the *Qi* in food into *Qi* can use. Then the Spleen Transports the *Qi* and Blood throughout the body.

- The Spleen governs Transportation and Transformation, transforms food into *Qi* and Blood; water transformation, which is "raising of the pure" for example raising the "pure" *Qi* to the Lungs, and raising "pure" thoughts.

- The Spleen also has the property of Distinguishing the "Five Tastes" that correspond to the five phases and is very important in herbology.

- The Spleen controls the Blood, this includes holding Blood in vessels; if you are always getting bruised OM would say your Spleen *Qi* must be deficient. The Spleen dominates the muscles and four limbs; the tone, texture, and strength of muscle is all Spleen related.

- The Spleen "Rules the Ascending"; the Spleen *Qi* ascends to the Lungs where it mixes with the air to begin the process of making Blood.

- General *Qi* Deficiency, or lethargy, or as the Chinese say "4 limbs heavy." This is where all of our limbs just seem heavy and hard to make move.

- Blood Deficiency: This is not a "classic syndrome" it is a secondary effect of Spleen Qi Deficiency. If the Spleen is not fully functioning it will impair the process of making Blood.

- Dampness: I'll give details later, but for now think of heaviness, dullness of mind, swelling, edema, overweight, excess mucous.

- Invasion from Liver: Caused from Liver *Qi* Stagnation, or from deficient Spleen *Qi*. If Spleen is weak it "invites" the Liver to invade.

As you can see the Spleen is involved in many of your bodies' processes, so the state of health or vitality of your Spleen will be very important in your overall state of health.

## Heart / Small Intestine

### HEART    Yin Organ

The Heart is also known as "The Supreme Ruler" or more commonly as the "Emperor." This is historically and clinically significant because of the understanding that the Ancient Chinese society had about their "Emperor" as being literally a manifestation of God in the physical plane. This understanding also stated that "there can be *nothing wrong* with the Emperor, as he is literally God-on-earth." So that meant that you could find no fault with the Heart or with a Heart Pulse. That also meant you could not treat anything dealing directly with the Heart meridian because that would imply there was something wrong with the Emperor, and trust me there is *never* anything wrong with the Emperor. His court officials may be corrupt, but the Emperor is *pure*.

So in a very pragmatic fashion, Oriental Medicine realized that the Pericardium was the "Protector of the Heart" and you could treat the physical ailments associated with the Heart by treating the Pericardium.

I find this to be very fascinating and very pragmatic. How did the Ancients know that the Pericardium was the protector of the Heart? And how did they know it would affect the physical ailments of the Heart?

The Heart's primary function is to govern the Blood and the Blood vessels and to "house the mind." Other Organ systems are also involved in governing the Blood, but the Heart is the primary Organ involved in circulation.

The term "housing the mind" is also interesting. In historical times it was seen as the Heart that was in control of the thinking and consciousness. The brain was largely not understood, though it was known if someone received a head injury their thinking could possibly be altered for life.

Oriental Medicine believes that the Heart "houses the *Shen*." The *Shen* is complex; it roughly corresponds to the mental faculties, but it also has the whole sphere of emotional, mental and spiritual aspects of a human being. Notice how many of the "duties" of the Heart have to do with mental-emotional considerations.

Maybe we should take this to say we should include our Heart in our thinking processes? I think we should, to a much greater degree than we currently do.

The Heart is associated with the Fire Phase, the color association is red, the season is Summer, the taste is bitter. Also, haven't we all heard of someone who has a 'bitter heart'? The emotion of the Heart is joy. Fire controls Metal so if the Fire is out of control it *may* manifest as mania that flashes over into grief; laughing then uncontrollably crying. The "insulting cycle" would be Fire attacking Water, very rare in Oriental Medicine but it does happen. The mania turning to paranoia…

One quick word about the emotion here; joy in and of itself is great. Where it becomes either an indicator of a deeper condition or of a problem in and of itself, is when there is excessive joy for no apparent reason. For example if I just lost my job and I am uncontrollably laughing and think this is the greatest thing that ever happened to me, that is an example of being out of balance or out of touch, with the deeper problem manifesting as excessive joy.

- The Heart opens to the Tongue; or said another way, the Tongue is seen as the "Sprout of the Heart." The Tongue is also seen as a "Mirror of Blood" ~ wherein the color of the Tongue reflects state of Heart and tongue.

- The Vitality of the Heart manifests in the complexion; if one's Heart is deficient your complexion will not be vibrant and healthy.

- The Heart dislikes Heat. Fright influences the Heart. Damp Heat in Liver from drinking alcohol leads to "Fire in Liver", which invades the Heart, making the face very Red.

- It is understood that the Heart controls Blood in the vessels.

- The Heart clarifies the Spirits *Hun* , *Shen, Yi, Po,* & *Jing* - See Chapter 14, page 149.

- The Heart Governs Blood and Blood Vessels; The Heart is the pump that circulates the blood throughout the body.

- The Heart Houses the *Shen* (Spirit): It is involved in all of these aspects of your life: mind, spirit, consciousness, memory, and thinking clearly.

- The Heart controls the ability to sleep: At night when it is time to sleep, it is understood that the Yang energy of the body comes to the Heart, where the Yin energy of the Heart Blood is to "embrace the Yang" and allow one to go to sleep. If the Yin is weak the Yang will never be able to settle down and sleep; or if the Yin is strong enough to allow the Yang to relax, but not strong enough to hold it, the Yang will 'pop free' and go wandering through the night, meaning you will wake up in the middle of the night and be awake for hours.

- The Heart Controls the Sweat: Heart *Qi* is very powerful. If the *Qi* of the Heart is injured, it may result in spontaneous sweating, and conversely if one sweats too much it may injure the Heart *Qi*. (Interestingly there is a correlation of this in Western medicine as well.)

- Dis-harmonies of the Heart may manifest as: madness; this can be anything from mild to extreme psychosis. Heart Blood deficiency may lead to restlessness and or insomnia, or forgetfulness.

I don't know about you, but **THIS IS GETTING TO BE WAY TOO SERIOUS.** So let's lighten things up a bit and give you something else to contemplate.

BlogPost: SUNDAY, NOVEMBER 19, 2006
## Almost Emergency Acupuncture
Yesterday while I was supervising at the school clinic I got a call from a woman that needed "emergency acupuncture" and wanted to see if we could fit her into the schedule. The clinic schedule was full, but I had an opening afterwards in my clinic. At 4 she came in with her husband.
She is a very thin, Hispanic lady, about 36 years old. She has severe asthma, and the asthma is causing panic attacks. She just got out of the hospital for an asthma-induced panic attack. She was breathing hard, and I could tell she was struggling just to keep it together. I told her and her husband I was going to do something I rarely, if ever do. Skip the intake process and just go to work. I only asked her to quantify her stress on that magical 1-10 scale. She put it at about a 12.
I get her comfortable on the table and start off with the treatment I jokingly call "Acuphoria" which is very calming and sedating; then I added in the auricular points to emphasize the calming effect.
We left the room to let her 'cook.'
I came back in the room in 10 minutes to check on her. She was very relaxed. After a total of 30 minutes her husband & I came back into the room to end the session. I was pleasantly surprised to see a smile on her face.

I was inspecting her ears to put some seeds in; you all know how impressed I am with their effectiveness. The area that corresponds to the "Heart" is so close to the "Lung" area that one piece of auricular tape and seed will cover both, and the tape is about 1/4" square. This entire area was red, which signals an imbalance.

When she got off the table I asked her what level her stress was at. She smiled and said about a 4. Not bad.

We are going to continue our work together; at best I just took one layer off. There is still a lot of work to do.

\*\*\*

OK, back to the current project, giving you all some useful information about Oriental Medicine.

## SMALL INTESTINES   Yang Organ

*Also known as the "Official in Charge of Separating the Pure from the Impure".*

The Primary function of the Small Intestine is to "Separate the Clear from the Turbid" in order to be able to send solid waste to the Large Intestine. The Small Intestine also sends liquid to Kidney and Bladder. The Small Intestines receive and temporarily store partially digested foods.

Heart & Small Intestine in Relationship: There is no simple way to put this, this is a dysfunctional relationship and it is hard to see the connection. One that does manifest is Heart Fire invades the Small Intestine, shown as ulcerations on tip of tongue, and blood in Urine.

***The five phase relationship is the same as for the Heart.***

I also find it interesting to note that the Small Intestine is also responsible for discernment, or sending pure information to the Emperor. With that in mind here is another blog post you might find interesting.

BlogPost: SUNDAY, MARCH 13, 2005

## The Power of Discernment

A few days ago I saw an interesting story on the national news; this young marine received two "purple-heart" medals resulting from injuries he received while in Iraq. One was a shrapnel wound, the other was a bullet that hit his right hand. This is the injury that got me thinking.

The bullet entered his right hand, just distal to the wrist, in the "knife-hand" area; the bullet penetrated through the palm of his hand just below the bones and exited from the web between his thumb and index finger.

Another way of saying this would be to say the bullet entered through SI-4 and exited from LI-4 area.

The young marine wants to return to Iraq; he feels he still has a mission to accomplish. I respect his intention, dedication, sacrifice and commitment. Yet his story has caused me to think about his injury. SI-4, Wangu translates as "wrist bone," no big surprise there. But what is interesting to me is one of my source books lists "improving discernment" as one of the Energetics of this point. I would have to acknowledge discernment has always been a tricky issue for me; sometimes I just do not know what the 'best' choice is. Maybe this is why I have been contemplating this injury. Anymore I just tend to look at it from the perspective of "Will this impede or improve my Spiritual Evolution?"

What I was thinking about concerning this young marine is, here he is with a major injury to this point and I am wondering, did this affect his ability to make a clear discernment concerning his future? Did the traumatic impact of that bullet slamming into Wangu affect his ability in a negative way, or in all fairness did it affect his discernment ability in a positive way, or not at all. Unless I knew him and was able to treat him I will never know. But it does raise an interesting point for contemplation.

The connection of LI-4, Hegu or "Joining Valley" is intriguing in that Hegu is also the "Command Point of the Head and Neck." This is primarily in regard to physical components; toothache, headache, stiff neck, these types of complaints.

Both Wangu and Hegu are Yuan-Source Points. The Yuan-Source Points are places where it is said that the Original (Yuan) Qi surfaces and lingers. The Yang Yuan-Source Points are used for treating excess conditions; they have a minimal 'tonifying' effect of their associated organ system complex.

So what happened to this young man's energy, his digestive tract, and even his cognition, his breathing and or sleeping? Small Intestine-4 is "paired" with the Heart; Large Intestine-4 is paired with the Lungs. The Heart is the Emperor and is where the Shen comes to rest at night in order for one to go to sleep. The Lungs house the "Corporeal Soul," one of five aspects of the Spirit. The emotion of the Lungs is "Grief;" the emotion of the Heart is "Joy." However I wonder; what about the bullet's impact? Does this young man have an inability to feel grief, or experience an inappropriate sense of joy? Is he experiencing insomnia? Has his digestion been affected? These are questions I would love to ask him. However, knowing me, I would ask him; "You want to return to Iraq? What are you thinking???"

\*\*\*

# Kidney / Urinary Bladder

## URINARY BLADDER   Yang Organ

The Urinary Bladder is known as the "District Official," or the minister in charge of the fluids of the body. The primary function of the Urinary Bladder is *Qi* Transformation ~ transforming and excreting fluids by the power of *Qi*; our bodies needs *Qi* to hold, transform and process fluids. As you can envision this is not a glorious job, but it is a necessary one, and this District Official does have some power bestowed upon it.

The Urinary Bladder receives the "dirty" part of fluids after the Small Intestine separates them from the "clean" fluids. The Urinary Bladder controls the storing of fluid and Directs *Qi* down.

Disharmony of the Urinary Bladder may manifest as:

### *Excess Patterns*

- Urinary Bladder Damp-Heat -- heat in urine, difficulty with urination, cloudiness of urine, short or scanty urine, dark urine or blood in urine.

- Urinary Bladder Damp-Cold -- light colored, copious urination

- Urinary Bladder obstructed by Turbid Heat -- more advanced Damp-Heat

- Heart Fire pours downward into Urinary Bladder

- General Symptoms of Excess: burning urine, insufficient & cloudy urine, headache (from back of head to top of head), olfactory problems, pain along spine or waist (Bladder Meridian), and or congestion in abdomen.

**Deficient Patterns**

- Urinary Bladder Deficient and Cold

General Symptoms of Deficiency: incontinence, frequent excessive urination, back pain, nocturnal enuresis, and fear.

- Kidney & Urinary Bladder in relationship: both mutually regulate water. Kidney is "Solid Organ" of Water, Urinary Bladder is "Hollow Organ" of Water.

Kidney Fire stokes Urinary Bladder. This is a 'good' type of Fire as we will see next.

Urinary Bladder Excess (*Fire*) leads to low back ache.

The U.B is associated with the Water Phase in the Five Phases, the color is black, the season is winter, and the taste is salty.

## KIDNEY   Yin Organ

The Kidneys are known as the "Strong Official from whom ingenuity derives." On the surface this is another of the enigmatic definitions that baffles us, but with a little explanation and investigation I think you will understand.

In Oriental Medicine the Kidney Organ system is essential. It is considered to be the root of *Qi*, the root of Life, and the Root of "Pre-heaven *Qi*" (What we were endowed with at the time of conception).

The Kidney opens to the ears; the ears are even shaped like kidneys. The Kidney is responsible for hearing, and difficulties with hearing.

The primary functions of the Kidney are: to "Store the *Jing*, the life essence" (this is the deepest aspect of 'who we are', it is our true Life Force, and our deepest Essence).

The kidneys are the foundation of Yin and Yang within the entire body. Kidney Yang controls the "ministerial fire," (what is called the "*Ming Men Huo*" or "Life Fire Door"). Kidney Yang also controls the Gate of Vitality of the Lower *Jiao*. (The word *Jiao* is translated as 'burner" or "opening")

The Kidney is the source of fire for all internal organs, especially the Spleen. There is a great drawing in one of my textbooks of an old fireplace/hearth. There is a decent sized fire in the hearth and there is a pot of stew hanging over the fire with steam coming off the stew. Keep that image in mind as you think of the functions/duties of the Kidney Organ system. If that fire is not big enough the stew will never get hot, if it is too big you could burn down the house or at least burn the stew.

The Kidney is associated with the Water Phase in the Five Phases, the color is black, the season is winter, and the taste is salty. The emotion of the Kidney is Fear. Water controls Fire, and the "insulting cycle" would have Water overflowing Earth.

Kidney Yin nourishes the Liver Yin and all other Yin in the body.

The Kidney Organ System is the root of Original *Qi*, and supplies Original *Qi* to all organs. The Kidney grasps and roots the *Qi* (Controls inhalation) If the Kidney is deficient it may not be able to reach up and grasp the *Qi* and root it in the body. If you experience 'shortness of breath" or 'breathlessness" and it is noticeably better when you lie down this is a good indication that the Kidney *Qi* is not grasping the Lung *Qi* to anchor your breath.

The Kidney rules the Bones. In OM the teeth are the excess of the bones. The Kidney produces Marrow (bone marrow, brain, spinal cord, and cerebral-spinal fluid) The Kidney is the "Root of Life"; it controls the entire life process. In OM men mature in 8 year cycles and women mature in 7 year cycles of birth, growth, maturation and death. The Kidney Organ system controls this process.

The Kidney dominates the water metabolism process; sending "pure" to the Lungs in a mist, and the turbid to the Urinary Bladder.

The Kidney warms the Lower *Jiao*. Kidney Yang *Qi* warms the

Uterus, as well as being the "pilot light" for the Spleen.

The Kidney is responsible for Heart balance; by this it is meant that the Kidney cools the Heart. Specifically, the Kidney Yin cools the *Heart*. The Kidney Organ system also assists the Heart in housing the *Shen* (the Spirit of YOU)

The Kidney controls the two "lower yin orifices", the anus and the urethra.

The Kidney directs *Qi* both up to the Spleen, and Lungs and down to the Urinary Bladder.

The Kidney produces feeling of awe and wonder, fear and apprehension, curiosity and vulnerability.

**Dis-harmony in the Kidney may manifest as:**

- Pain, discomfort or sensitivity. Tension or abnormal sensations may be felt spontaneously or elicited upon palpation in the lumbar region, the waist, the loins, pelvic area, and or the vicinity of the $12^{th}$ rib. It is understood that the Kidney rules the lower back.

- Low Back Pain, including knee pain, weak ankles, and sciatic nerve pain.

- Impotence and infertility are primary indicators of Kidney disharmony and or deficiency.

This list also includes: incontinence (urinary, or seminal), urinary frequency, loss of hearing including deafness, tinnitus, (as well as other hearing issues), chronic loose stools (especially in early morning hours), problems of growth and development, premature signs of aging including premature hair loss, loss of hearing, eyesight, loss of teeth. Edema must be included; but with other Organ systems. Facial edema indicates Lungs, abdominal edema indicates Spleen, and edema in the lower extremities indicates Kidneys. (Accumulation of adipose tissue is usually Dampness)

- The Kidney is "strained" by overwork, is "drained" by too much of the salty flavor, and is "overwhelmed" by excessive fear.

- The Kidney is exhausted by too much sexual activity especially orgasms/childbirth and or abortions.

Kidney Excess Patterns: <u>The Kidney is rarely, if ever, in excess</u>.

*Kidney Deficiency Patterns:*

- Kidney Jing Deficiency (impotence or infertility), Kidney failing to grasp Qi is seen as a shortness of breath that is relieved when you lay down.

- Kidney Yang Deficiency manifests as Qi Deficiency with Cold signs; Kidney Yang deficiency with Water Overflowing. This can lead to what is known in Western medical terms as "congestive heart failure".

- Kidney Yin deficiency manifesting as frequent short urination, low back pain, and excessive (relative) heat.

General signs of Kidney Deficiency: indecisiveness, confused speech, dreams of trees submerged under water Classic dream interpretation and who ever heard of this???, cold feet and legs, abundant sweating, fearfulness deep fears, "real" fear, apathy, discouragement, scatteredness, lack of will, negativity, impatience, low sex drive, lumbago and or sciatica.

As you can see from all this information, the Kidney Organ system is integral to your overall health. We all tend to over-tax our Kidney's which tends to damage our health through these inadvertent activities.

# Pericardium / San Jiao

### PERICARDIUM Yin Organ

The Pericardium is known as the official that protects the Heart, or the minister who insulates, screens and protects. The Pericardium maintains the order of the Heart energy.

Remember in historical China one could not say there was anything 'wrong' with the Heart, as the Heart was seen as the Emperor and we all know there is nothing wrong with the Emperor -- ever.

So it has evolved over the centuries that one can now use the Heart points and meridian to treat the "Spiritual" aspect of the

'Heart Energetics', and use the Pericardium to treat the actions of the Heart. It is said one will "Treat the Heart through the Pericardium."

The primary function of the Pericardium is to protect the Heart; it is the last line of defense for the Heart. The Pericardium receives "evil pathogens" before it reaches the heart. This is very similar to one of the functions of the pericardium in Western medicine.

The Pericardium also confers sense of speech through its sense organ ~ the tongue.

The Pericardium controls the vascular system, including the Blood, Pulse & Special tissue of the heart.

By "Treat the Heart through the Pericardium" it is meant to be able to treat the Organic Function of Heart (palpitations for example). Yet to treat a "Spirit" imbalance one can treat Heart *or* Pericardium.

The Pericardium is seen as the Origin of Joy & Sadness; it produces feelings of Joy and Pleasure.

The Pericardium dislikes Heat, the same as the Heart.

Healthy expressions for the Pericardium are Joy, Happiness, and Healthy Relationships.

The Pericardium has such a close relationship with the Heart it too is associated with the Fire Phase, the color association is red, the season is Summer, the taste is bitter and the emotion is joy.

***Dis-harmony of the Pericardium may manifest as:***

- Pain, discomfort, or abnormal sensations usually experienced in the Chest.

- Sensitivity and/or Tension can often be palpated in the mid-sternal area (the middle of the breastbone).

Other signs may include confusion, delirium, nervous energy and or sexual perversions.

The Pericardium may be adversely affected by: Emotional Stresses internally, or Invasion of Heat externally. These two causes can be from a hectic hurried lifestyle. This can also be caused by "Excessive use of the Eyes", which is overstimulation; watching TV for hours, then playing computer games etc., etc. You get the idea; modern life in America. This is also seen as too much excitement, which may lead to hysteria. These effects are usually very pronounced in children.

## SAN JIAO   Yang Organ

Here is an Organ System with which there is NO Western medical or scientific corollary. The "*San Jiao*" is literally translated as "three burners"; this Organ System is truly an "Energetic phenomenon", not an organ system as we would normally think of one.

The "Three Burners" or "Triple Heater" are three divisions within the abdominal cavity. The "Lower Burner" or Lower *Jiao* is from the pelvic floor up to about your navel. The "middle Burner" or Middle *Jiao* is from about your navel to your diaphragm right at the bottom of your rib cage. And the "Upper Burner" or Upper *Jiao* is from the diaphragm to the top of your lungs.

Each of the three *Jiao*'s have specific functions, and they all interact with each other to fulfill their functions.

The *San Jiao* simultaneously monitors and regulates the Internal environment to maintain optimal operating temperatures. It is said that the Yang of the *San Jiao* Metabolic process is like a "Fire" that provides heat with which to process materials and energy; whereas the Yin of the *San Jiao* is "Water." Among other functions this is an important means of heat dissipation to keep the system from overheating.

The *San Jiao* is the official in charge of Irrigation; this is Classically defined as a System of Sluices or Waterways - the form of the water is different in each.

Upper Jiao = Mist/Fog (Water vapor)

Middle Jiao = Foam (Gruel)

Lower Jiao = Swamp/Dregs (Wastewater)

One of my favorite saying is "*The San Jiao has a name but has NO FORM*"; by this it is meant there is no "*San Jiao* Organ", it is entirely an Energetic system. The *San Jiao* is "function without substance", the *San Jiao* is like Yin/Yang in that Yin/Yang has function but no substance either. There is no physical substrate. Another way to think of this is the Three *Jiao*'s roughly correspond to our notion of metabolism (Catabolism and Anabolism).

The *San Jiao* is also seen as an "envelope that protects the *Shen* (Spirit) from outside evils." According to one of my favorite authors, Kiko Matasumoto; "the *San Jiao* = Immune Function."

*The San Jiao is a Pathway of Fluids*: the Upper *Jiao* water is a "Mist" in the Lungs; the Middle *Jiao* water is "Foam" in the Stomach / Spleen, and the Lower *Jiao* water is like a "Swamp" in the Kidneys / Bladder / Large Intestine / Small Intestine

Or stated another way the Upper *Jiao* houses the Lungs, which adjust water, The Middle *Jiao* houses the Spleen which transforms water If the Spleen is not able to transform water it will stagnate and turn into Phlegm, and the Lower *Jiao* houses the Kidneys, which rule water.

The *San Jiao* is also reflected in the Pulse: The three positions of the pulse are said to reflect the three *Jiao*'s. The most distal (closest to your wrist) position relates to the upper warmer, the farthest from your wrist (closer to your elbow) reflects the lower warmer.

The *San Jiao* communicates with all organs to help them work together. I see the *San Jiao* also as a "communication matrix" that facilitates the communication process of the organs.

A definition of health modeled on *San Jiao* Principles: Health is the ability of an organism to respond or adapt appropriately to an ever changing environment. This is accomplished by constant adjustment to the demands of the external environment.

Adaptability ~ Physiological, Psychological, Emotional, and Spiritual. This adaptability requires very precise, yet dynamic heat regulation. Our bodies have a continual feedback system where the end product is known as Homeostasis -- though I think of it as "Homeodynamism." Homeostatic regulation keeps the body operating optimally. Oriental Medicine names this function in all its many aspects the *"San Jiao."*

As Jim, one of my teachers says "This is all very interesting, but what do you do with it?"

## Liver / Gallbladder

### GALLBLADDER     Yang Organ

The Gallbladder is also known as "The Official in Charge of Decision making". One author refers to the Gallbladder as the "Master at Arms".

The Gallbladder is responsible for decision making; and the source of courage and initiative.

The Gallbladder is an "extraordinary" hollow Organ in that it stores a pure substance, the bile that was secreted by the Liver. The Liver excretes the bile, which is not normal for a solid organ, and the Gallbladder stores the bile --to be sent to the Small Intestine, which is then used in digestion / transformation-- which is unusual for a hollow organ.

Another way that the Gallbladder is 'extraordinary' for a Yang Organ is that the Gallbladder is said to have an emotion expressed through it. So far whenever I have said an Organ System has an emotional component it has always been a Yin, or a "Solid" Organ System. Just as there are always exceptions to the rules, there is an exception to this pattern as well. The Gallbladder expresses the emotion of resentment. So in this too, the Gallbladder is close to the Liver. Anger and resentment are very interrelated.

The Gallbladder is very closely related to the Liver. Sometimes this is referred to as LiverGallbladder.

The primary function of the Gallbladder is to purify Yang energy in the body. The Yang energy needs to be clear, or pure to rise to the head.

The Gallbladder is responsible for decision making; it is the source of courage and initiative. The Liver makes the plans, but the Gallbladder is the source of the courage to make the decisions and act on the plans.

The Gallbladder, with the Liver, controls the sense of sight through its sense organ, the Eyes.

The Gallbladder dislikes "Wind"

Dis-harmonies of the Gallbladder may manifest with these General Symptoms:

- Rash angry decisions, a lateral headache affecting primarily the sides of your head, muscular spasms, limbs slightly cold, heaviness in head and stomach (a symptom of the Yang $Qi$ not being purified and rising to the head), a bitter taste in mouth (also a "Classic" Liver symptom), jaundice, vomiting bitter fluid, and/or nausea.

*Gallbladder Deficiency Patterns:*

- Indecisiveness, and or Timidity (both of these are "Classic" Gallbladder Deficiency Symptoms), cowardice, frustration, irritability, and/or depression.

*The Liver & Gallbladder in Relationship:*

It is said that the Gallbladder resides in the Liver, this is one way of describing that their relationship is very close. They assist one another in decision making, and appropriate responses.

## LIVER     Yin Organ

Liver is also known as "The Official in Charge of Planning." The Liver is also known as "The General" who plans or coordinates. The Liver is sometimes known as the "Free and Easy Wanderer, being gentle and laid back." The Free and Easy Wanderer "sprinkles *Qi*" and maintains an easy going environment.

The Liver opens to the Eyes, the Liver dislikes Wind, also Heat/Stagnation

The Liver is said to have the properties of: Flowing and Spreading; this is to say that the Qi of the Liver is intended to flow throughout the body and to spread through all Organ systems. Or stated another way the Liver regulates the harmonious distribution of *Qi* throughout the body (even-flowing, uniform spreading of *Qi*)

I do think of the Liver as the "General". The way that I would talk about the Liver is this, "Each Organ system is likened to a court official, and the Liver is said to be the General. When I think about a general, one way I see this is that a General wants to be able to go anywhere, at any time, with no questions asked. If you tell a General that he cannot go somewhere, he gets mad. Now as we all know, a General will attack another army; but a good general will not attack a stronger army. He will look around and find an army he can beat. In our body this manifests as the Liver *Qi* not being able to flow freely which causes the Liver to get *mad*. Then the Liver looks around and finds an Organ system that is weak and attacks it. It is very common for the Liver to attack the Stomach. You may experience this as first you get mad, and then you get a stomachache."

The Liver directs *Qi* uniformly in all directions; it is said that the Liver "sprinkles the *Qi*" meaning it spreads or disperses the *Qi* throughout our body.

The Liver harmonizes the emotions so that what we are feeling is appropriate for the situation and is expressed appropriately.

The Liver regulates the menses, in particular the menstrual cycle is controlled by the Liver, the amount of menses is controlled by the Spleen.

The Liver regulates the normal function of the body and promotes function of all organ systems.

**The Liver Rules the Muscles**

The Liver governs the motor system: controls mobility, and voluntary muscle system.

The Liver regulates the ability of muscles to contract. Liver Wind can cause contraction of muscles. The Liver is responsible for the moistening of ligaments and tendons; which, if out of balance, could lead to an inability to flex freely, and dry ligaments and tendons causes muscular spasms.

The Liver houses the ethereal soul, the persona, the ego.

**The Liver Stores the Blood.**

The Liver nourishes the eyes. Liver Blood Deficiency = dry eyes and or blurred vision; or dry, rough feeling eyes. In Oriental Medicine, seeing "Floaters" (those little spots that are within our eyes, but tend to move around when we blink) is seen as being directly correlated to the Liver Blood Deficiency.

The Liver nourishes the menses, so for nearly all menstrual irregularities there will be some degree of Liver involvement.

It is said that the condition of the Liver is observable in the nails, and that the Liver controls the eyes and "opens to the eyes."

The liver is also involved in our "mental vision" or how we can visualize internally. The Liver also controls, or at least contributes to our mental outlook.

When in dis-harmony the Liver produces feelings of anger, frustration, irritability, and depression.

The Liver is "strained" by overuse of the eyes, and or overuse of the musculoskeletal system (Overwork, and or over-exercise… Remember, a little bit of something is good, too much of something is bad…)

The Liver is "drained" by too much sour, astringent flavor; and the Liver is "overwhelmed" by excessive rage, too much frustration.

**Dis-harmonies of the Liver may manifest as:**

- Liver Qi Stagnation is the primary dis-harmony and it has many faces.

- Invading the Stomach. The way I look at this is the General gets angry when stagnated, and strikes out. (If an organ is weak it "invites" an invasion. If the General is angry he does not look for a strong organ to invade.) Liver stagnation may manifest as a hiatal hernia, where the stomach "pops through" the upper diaphragm, causing sharp stabbing intense pain. Or as heartburn, or ulcers, acid reflux, or even vomiting.

- Invading the Spleen, which may manifest as irritable bowels, Crohn's disease (passing blood and mucous)

- Invading the Lungs; which may manifest as stress-induced asthma, or crying when very angry.

- "Plum-Pit stuck in the throat" This is a literal description of the feeling; that causes constant throat clearing.

**Liver Excess Patterns:**

- Liver & Gallbladder are invaded by damp heat; this can manifests in two ways. In the Meridian; the signs are along the meridian. Herpes Zoster (Shingles) appears on the Gallbladder Meridian. Or Jaundice with an "orange" twinge to the face. "Hot Jaundice" has orange as a base color.

- "Liver Fire Blazing Upwards": This is where the Liver Stagnation generates fire. Some people experience violent headaches at the top of their head, leading to violent outbursts. I know of one man that first gets angry, then a 'raging headache' at the top of his head and if it is not 'caught' can get physically violent directly after the headache 'peaks.'

- "Liver Invaded by Cold Damp": "Cold Jaundice" which manifests' as a sallow, or pale yellow face color.

- "Liver Invading Spleen" or "Liver Invading Stomach" which manifests first as anger/frustration that leads to a stomachache and or stomach cramps.

- "Liver Meridian Obstructed by Stagnant Cold" which could manifest as lumps on external genitalia, or "Cold Lumps" in lower abdomen. Also lumps in breast tissues could be Liver related.

- "Mild Liver Qi Stagnation" will manifest with mild problems: soreness, anger. Mildness is the key.

- "Liver Wind arising from Liver Yang Rising" or "Liver Wind Stirring". This is internally generated; shakes, Parkinson's disease, Tourette's syndrome. One thing to ponder: Are seizures Liver winds raging out of control?

- "Liver Yang Rising" This is described as having symptoms halfway between Liver Qi Stagnation and Liver Fire Blazing upwards. The progression appears to be Liver Qi Stagnation, which, if left untreated can change to Liver Yang Rising. If left untreated, this can change to Liver Fire Blazing Upwards.

### General symptoms of Liver Qi Excess

Excessive muscular tension, excitability, red tearing eyes, insomnia, compulsive energy, moodiness and or a bitter taste in mouth (This is "The Classic" symptom in Oriental Medicine, but it may not always be experienced.)

**Liver Blood Patterns: Liver Blood Deficiency, Liver Blood Stagnation, Liver Yin Deficiency, and Liver Wind Arising from Liver Blood Deficiency**

**General Liver Blood Symptoms:**

Weakness in muscles and tendons, especially of the legs, difficulty standing and walking, vertigo (sense of room spinning), which is different than dizziness, (which is an impaired sense of balance, but not the room spinning), insomnia can be Liver Yin Deficiency (causing an inability to sleep) <u>excessive sighing</u>, which is a combination of deficiency and stagnation.

**Gynecological Problems:**

- Menstrual Problems: especially symptoms of PMS, breast pain and distention, dysmenorrhia: in particular having painful periods may be Liver *Qi* Stagnation, uterine bleeding, abnormal flow (scanty or heavy) Also remember that if the Spleen is not producing Blood, flow will be scanty; if the Liver is not storing, the flow will be heavy.

From this description you can see why the "general" has an attitude; he is responsible for a lot of things and it always seems as though something is out of balance. After a while he just gets angry…

**OH MY GOSH THAT WAS A LOT OF INFORMATION.**

## FROM HERE IT WILL BE EASIER.

Just a few closing thoughts on Organ Systems; it is important to remember that when an Oriental Medical practitioner mentions an Organ he or she is NOT talking about your Western organ system unless they say they are. For example I may be treating someone with Hepatitis C and we will be having a multi-paradigm discussion about their liver, and their Liver. Both the organ and the Organ will be involved in the discussion, understanding and treatment protocol.

If you are unclear whether your OM practitioner is talking about the OM understanding of the Organ or the Western understanding of the organ, just ask them. It is important for you to understand all facets of your health care.

Finally even though I wrote out many confusing and or conflicting descriptions of different Organs systems do not get too complicated in your thinking about them. In general if you tonify the Spleen and Kidneys and "Course" (move) the Liver *Qi* many of the symptoms one is experiencing will start to balance. All of the Organs are connected and or related in some way, so by tonifying the Kidneys and Spleen it will help all of the other Organs. By 'Coursing' the Liver *Qi* it will reduce Stagnation and allow the Liver to nourish all of the body.

Again a bit of repetition, but another way of looking at concepts...

BlogPost: TUESDAY, FEBRUARY 15, 2005

## Boundaries: A Function of the San Jiao Meridian?

This week I have been thinking of the San Jiao Meridian. The San Jiao is unique in many ways, but the most intriguing concept is that is does not have an organ system complex associated with it in the same manner as the other meridians. There is a physical substrate for the Heart, Lungs Spleen, etc., but not so with the San Jiao.

The name San Jiao translates as the "Three Openings;" a reference to the three 'burner's'. The Nan Jing, an ancient classical text, refers to the San Jiao as "having a name, but no form." Instead the Nan Jing seems to attribute the functions of water metabolism to the San Jiao, it is said that the "Upper Jiao is like a mist, the middle Jiao is like foam and the lower Jiao is like a sluiceway." In Chinese medical theory the San Jiao is integral to the transformation of qi and the free flow of fluids throughout.

The San Jiao is also used, clinically, to diagnose externally contracted febrile disease. By accurately assessing how deep the pathogen has penetrated, the practitioner will determine the course of treatment. The upper burner (Lungs) is the first to be affected and the lower burner (Kidneys) is a more serious condition. Using the upper, middle or lower burner as a classification for the disease 'center' is useful, but in the clearest of definitions that is not a "San Jiao" classification, remember the San Jiao has a name, but no form. It does give the practitioner a practical way of addressing the condition, though not through the San Jiao meridian.

As an example let's say a patient has digestive problems, loose stools, fatigue after eating, bruises easily, his tongue is pale and scalloped. In TCM this is a very simplified pattern of Spleen Qi Deficiency. One could also say the middle burner, or middle Jiao is affected. But the treatment would not be focused on the San Jiao. Of course, I want to look at it in a slightly different light.

Let's also say that same patient has been working in a job that he truly does not enjoy, the work environment is demeaning to him but he is keeping the job because in another 18 years he can retire from it. You might say he is having trouble digesting that choice.

I also think of the San Jiao as being integral to one's boundary system. Boundaries are important not only in the physical sense, how close do I let someone get to me (physically, emotionally, and spiritually) but also in a less concrete manner. Do I allow the words that someone else says to enter and lodge into my belief system? Do I believe what others may or may not be saying about me? I think that the ability to process and function as one navigates the maze of determining what to let in and what to throw out is a function of the San Jiao.

For this discussion it is also important to recognize the interior/exterior paired meridian complex, the Pericardium. In TCM the Pericardium is the "Heart Protector," its function is seen literally as protecting the Heart from evil pathogens. The question then becomes what is the difference between an "evil pathogen" and an unhealthy thought pattern that affects the way you see yourself in the world? Or stated another way, if the Yang aspect of this interior/exterior paired meridian, the San Jiao, does not function at its strongest it will allow the unhealthy thought to penetrate into your beingness and then it is the job of the Pericardium to protect your Heart from the inclusion of that thought into your world view.

Now, back to our patient. If this man can choose to look at how his choice of staying at a job he does not like is affecting his health he might be able to determine if the cost (poor health that most likely will deteriorate) is worth the reward ("retirement" IF all things go as planned and the company does not close or out-source his job).

So part of the treatment might very well include San Jiao concepts as I am seeing them, but only if the patient desires to get into that depth of being. As I wrote about in a previous blog, if one is following his or her destiny the payoff for that is good health and a longer life. Who am I to decide that for a patient? Yet I also have an obligation to open the door to this type of a conversation and see if he or she is willing to enter into this type of a discussion.

The concept of the San Jiao is intriguing to me. Having a name, but no form, not being associated with a physical substrate organ, being paired with the Heart Protector; all of that is one of the interesting paradoxes of Chinese medicine. I am not sure if any of this will make sense to anyone that ever reads it, but it is an interesting perspective to consider. If you like it, great. If not, in the words of Bruce Lee "Pare away the unnecessary."

***

# Chapter 10

# "Got Fire?"

When I was first learning about Oriental Medicine and I heard the term "Fire" I thought to myself "what the heck are they talking about?" I knew that we did not have "Fire" in our bodies. I may have been born at night, but I was not born last night.

It took a while for it to penetrate my mind that the phrase does not mean the literal manifestation. Then I started to think maybe the term was used to describe the metabolic or digestive processes. I was a little closer, but still off the mark.

As mentioned earlier, I see the 'temperature continuum" as going from cold to cool to neutral to warm to hot and finally to fire. As you can see from that example Fire is at the far end of the range. As with most extremes in life, it is an area to avoid if possible.

There are two very simple ways of experiencing "Fire;" one is to have too much heat, the other is to have too little cooling; or said another way, too much Yang, or too little Yin. Both will manifest as Fire, but will have a totally different "root cause". As mentioned earlier, you will not get the best results if you do not treat the root cause correctly.

Too much Yang, or too much Heat does happen, though not as frequently as too little Yin. Here the usual cause would be too much hot spicy foods and/or liquor. Both hot spicy foods and liquor instill or create heat in your body. After a time your body may say "enough is enough." Then again you may be one of those people that can eat habanero peppers without breaking a sweat. Most of us cannot do that, or if we do we will pay for it later.

Once your body has generated more Heat than it can process or tolerate, you will start to develop certain signs and symptoms: a higher level of thirst, your tongue may be a deeper shade of red than before, or it may have "prickles" on the tongue body; your pulse may be more rapid than normal.

Too little Yin or cooling will have different signs and symptoms. This condition is also called "Empty Heat" because it is actually from a deficiency.

When there is a Yin Deficiency some very common signs are:

a low-grade fever or a feeling of heat in the afternoon, what is called "5 palm heat" (heat in the soles of your feet, the palms of your hands and the center of your chest), a dry throat at night and or night-sweats. As you ladies that have gone through 'the change of life' know, this sounds very familiar.

A simple comparison between Excess or Full Heat and Deficient or Empty Heat

| Excess / Full Heat | Deficient / Empty Heat |
|---|---|
| Fever any time, day or night | PM Fever warm in the afternoons. PM Hot flashes |
| Thirst wants a lot of water, cool to cold water | Dry mouth sips water, but not really thirsty |
| Sore throat | Chronic dry / scratchy throat Chronic non- productive cough |
| Red face, red eyes | Flush cheeks |
| Constipation, hot diarrhea | Dry stools |
| Dark burning scanty urine | Dark scanty urine |
| Pulse: rapid, full | Pulse: thin empty, rapid |

**Heat / Fire**

Signs and Symptoms:

- Aversion to cold, which is counter-intuitive but empirically accurate, shivering, sneezing, cough, runny nose with yellow mucous (heat is drying out mucous)

- Fever predominates over chills, slight stiffness / body ache, a slight sweat, restlessness, (thirst because the Heat is frying out fluids), and or a sore scratchy throat

- Pulse: floating, rapid

- Tongue: Red Tip / Sides, slight yellow or white tongue coat

**Fire**

Fire is more solid, more "hot" than heat.

Fire has more substance, and does more damage than just heat.

Fire injures Blood and Yin. Fire is usually internal. Fire moves upward. Fire can cause pain; Fire causes ulcers, and boils.

Fire Affects the Mind causing anxiety, agitation, insomnia, and or psychosis. When someone has a "Liver Yang Rising" type of headache the most prevalent symptom is the headache starts at the very top of their head. It may spread to other parts of their head, but it almost always starts at the top.

Fire can cause bleeding, this is a most serious condition, it can result in death. This is because Fire agitates the Blood; when this happens the Blood may be in cough, vomit, stools, urine, or irregularity of menses. In severe cases the Blood will leave the blood vessels and be just under the skin.

Fire can be *Shi* (True excess heat) or *Xu* (False "excess" heat). The symptoms are different, and because the root cause is different the treatment must also be different.

# Chapter 11

# "You Be Damp!"

"Dampness" is that extra cushion of adipose (fat) tissue, water, or phlegm. Dampness as seen and understood by Oriental Medicine is caused by internal or external conditions. Internally if your Spleen is not fully transforming the foods you eat the excess will be stored as dampness. If it is stored for a long time, and or you have excess Heat it will turn into Phlegm. This is important because "All strange diseases come from phlegm."

Externally generated dampness, living in wet areas hot humid and or swampy, will have a penetrating effect and this will over time bypass your defensive *Qi* and enter into your body.

Signs and symptoms of Dampness are sweating without exertion or moist skin; musculoskeletal stiffness which is due to joints being more full or swelling; a heavy feeling throughout your body and or heavy lingering pain

The one thing I always try to impart to someone with Dampness is that your diet has an enormous effect on this. In the recommended reading you will find the information on a couple of good nutritionally sound books. Investigate and see what combination works best for you.

As I mentioned all strange diseases are said to come from Phlegm. Phlegm can be thought of, in our simplistic way, as coming from

Dampness. Strange diseases are any dis-ease that defies treatment, or has multiple complicated symptoms.

Also, your diet is one of, if not *the* single most impacting decision you make every day. Food is medicine, and food can be poison. These conditions do not appear overnight, it is from years of poor dietary decisions that one generates a 'strange disease.'

## Phlegm Vs Damp

| **Phlegm / Dilute Phlegm** | **Damp / Water** |
|---|---|
| Only Internal causes | External or Internal causes |
| Spleen, Lung and Kidney involved | Spleen responsible |
| Affects mostly Yin Organs Lungs, Heart, Kidney & Spleen Upper and middle primarily, but can go and affect any area of the body. | Affects mostly yang organs Liver, Large Intestine, & Stomach Heavy, dirty, turbid, sinking… Mainly affects the lower Can also prevent the rising of Clear Yang |
| Feelings of cloudiness and dizziness | Feeling of heaviness |
| Affects the mental functions | No effect on the mental functions |
| Congealed: Moveable lumps and nodules, some joint deformities | Affects the joints (swelling) |
| Tongue: thick, sticky, prickles, hairs, dry, rough (esp. in Stomach area) | Tongue: thin, sticky coat May be slippery |
| Pulse: Slippery, possibly wiry | Pulse: Slippery |
| Combines with: Wind, Heat, Cold, Damp, *Qi* | Combines With: Heat, Cold, Wind, Water |

# Part Four

# Chapter 12

# "We Don't Treat Disease!"

BlogPost: TUESDAY, NOVEMBER 22, 2005

**It is bound to happen**

Today I am pondering the impact of practicing medicine when a friend's health is being impacted. Today one of my patients came in and told me she is waiting on the results of a breast biopsy. She has a genetic prevalence towards breast cancer and her yearly mammogram has some areas of concern. The biopsy was last Thursday and the results will be told to her later this morning.

I am realizing many things as I write this. First of all I am seeing the potential for how cancer can impact any one's life so suddenly. I do not believe that she has cancer, but I may be wrong. But I am also thinking of a good friend and classmate that is dealing with breast cancer. It feels to me like everyone's life, on one level or another, is being impacted by cancer. Do you know of anyone that does not know someone that is dealing with some form of cancer?

I am also realizing how allopathic medicine treats cancer and I see, immediately, my bias coming into focus. I do not think that we have to "Fight" cancer, I think there can be a way to work with the cancer and to minimize its impact.

I am also remembering the saying that "There can be a healing without a cure and but there is not a true cure without a healing." If one's lifestyle has created the dis-ease how can there be a cure (resolution of the dis-ease) without a healing (awareness of the latent cause of the dis-ease)? In that case, (a cure without a healing) it seems to me that the dis-ease will return. Maybe in a different manner or presentation, but I believe it will return. Conversely, if there is a 'healing' it does not matter as much if there is a cure. There are some things worse than death.

The incidence of cancer in our society is significant. One hundred years ago it was not as prevalent, but in truth we did not have the diagnostic abilities that we do now so it may have been somewhat higher than we understand it to have been. Nonetheless the incidence of cancer is significantly higher than historical levels.

Would I be going TOO FAR OUT ON A LIMB to say that I believe this is because of three or four significant "technological advances" that have occurred within our time.

1) The use and or overuse of chemicals. The food chain is saturated with chemicals. We are all eating these chemicals and worse yet cooking them which significantly alters their composition.

2) The use of growth hormones. I could write a book on this one, but suffice it to say that a substance that makes cows and chickens grow bigger and fatter IS going to alter our bodies natural growth and maturation process. When that natural cycle is altered and out of balance cancer has an open door to sneak in through.

3) Electromagnetic fields. We are, on one level, an electromagnetic field. When our 'field' is constantly being bombarded with other, much higher powered EMF's it has to, on some level, affect our intrinsic electromagnetic field.

4) Microwave energy. Aside from cooking with a microwave (which depletes the qi from the food you are going to eat) we are all being bombarded by microwaves, TV towers, Cell phone towers, and satellite communications. The list goes on, but this is an extremely high powered form of energy. If it can boil water, you know it can cook you as well.

So I would love to hear from any of you about your thoughts on this. Am I reading dread into nothing? Am I just freaked out because of a set of coincidences? What do you think???

By the way, my friend/patient called in and reported the biopsy is clean. AT LEAST THAT IS SOME GOOD NEWS TO BE THANKFUL FOR.

***

So a lot of the times by the time someone comes into an acupuncturist's office he or she is at, or near the end, of their rope, so to speak. Usually a patient will have been to nearly every doctor they can think of or afford to try. Many times the condition that they are seeking help for will have been a part of their life for over a decade.

My primary martial arts teacher used to tell us, "Listen to the whispers, and avoid hearing the shouts." I think this is very sound advice.

We are all able to learn from and listen to our bodies; our bodies are filled with an innate wisdom. As an acupuncturist I have to be able to learn to listen to your body as well. Luckily for all of us the language is pretty simple.

If an Oriental Medical practitioner is well trained he or she can pick up on many subtle imbalances before they manifest at a clinical level. We can learn what is 'normal' for your body and then if that starts to change we can address it before it becomes an issue.

That is all well and fine if you are receiving acupuncture treatments on a regular basis, but as I said most patients come in for a treatment when things are already out of balance and have been for a number of years. By this point you may very well have a condition that is named. "You have Crohn's Disease." "You have Irritable Bowel Syndrome" or "You have Endometriosis."

There are several things I want you to understand about this. First off, when a western doctor pronounces you with a "disease" I feel it is very important to understand that this label may, or may not include an understanding of the *underlying causes* of the condition.

As I mentioned at the beginning of this book, Western Medicine is extremely powerful, and there are many, many cases where if you want to live, you need Western Medicine. If I get in a car wreck, send me to a hospital, thank you very much! But as soon as I am stable, I will be changing my medical treatments.

Western Medicine is very strong at treating symptoms; but it is conversely, in my opinion at least, noticeably weaker in addressing the underlying causes of those symptoms.

So you may be able to get the symptoms somewhat under control, but they may come back despite your best effort. Or maybe you can get them under control, but the side effects of the medicine are horrible and have a severely negative impact on the quality of your life. You may bounce around from one doctor to another, one treatment system to another. Time goes on and you find yourself asking "Am I getting any better for all this time, effort and money I am spending on this?

Then, out of desperation, you go into an acupuncturist's office thinking "I have tried everything else, I might as well give this a try." (I have had patients actually tell me those exact words.) Then your acupuncturist tells you "I am sorry to tell you this, but acupuncture does not treat disease."

"Excuse me, *what did you say*?"

What your acupuncturist will then explain is how Oriental Medicine looks at the body, health and balance. He or she will explain that yes, we can treat the symptoms that are causing you such grief, but we will be going deeper into searching out and rectifying the 'root cause' of the imbalance. She or he will then try to help you understand that your body did not get into this state of imbalance overnight most likely and it will take a reasonable amount of time to return to a normal balance and state of health.

A few paragraphs back I mentioned an old saying I was taught. "Learn to listen to the whispers and avoid hearing the shouts." It seems we are missing something in our normal health education. Learning to listen to the whispers does take time and effort. We are all bombarded with stimulus all the time; in fact I think we can even become addicted to stimulation. But my point is that when there is this much stimulation impacting our consciousness all the time it is hard to 'unplug' and learn to listen to the 'small quiet voice within.' But the result is priceless.

Our bodies can tell us if a certain food is good for us, neutral or bad for us. I know someone who loves chocolate, and she knows she has to be careful of what is in the chocolate or she will have a reaction to it. She can have a piece of chocolate in her hand and if she is going to react to it she will start sneezing within 10 seconds of holding on to this chocolate. Your body will tell you this type of information if you will take the time to learn to listen to it.

When you learn to listen to and respect what your body is telling you, you can avoid hearing the shouts. The shouts manifests as "disease," literally dis-ease.

By learning to listen to the subtle lessons of the foods we eat, we can return to our natural state of health more easily. When we learn to trust our bodies we can learn whether or not we can be exposed to the electromagnetic forces of a computer screen for hours without health consequences. This same learning can also be applied to discerning what are the internal effects of being a witness to a violent act; as it DOES have an effect on everyone that witnesses one. I know that we can learn to become aware of what our bodies already know but has escaped our mental awareness. I also have to wonder if maybe we have just been deluded through the mainstream media. Who knows?

BlogPost: THURSDAY, APRIL 14, 2005

## It just goes to show

I had the honor a few weeks ago of giving a treatment to a truly world-class athlete. I have asked her permission to write about this, because it is so amazing to me.
Pam Reed just completed a world-record 300 mile no-sleep run. She took just under 80 hours to complete this amazing feat. Imagine starting at 6:00 a.m. Friday morning and running without stop-

ping for sleep until Monday at 2 in the afternoon. Just the accomplishment is nearly unbelievable. If I hadn't been with her for part of the time I would have wondered about her cognitive faculties towards the end of the run. I was lucky enough to spend Sunday night from 8 until 5 Monday morning riding my bike next to her. She was lucid and able to converse. At about 2 a.m. she got quiet, but never slowed down or stopped her run. I was giving her leg massages at the end of a lap (25 miles). All of this is amazing and was a pleasure to be around. That kind of dedication and perseverance is always inspiring.

But of course that is not what I am truly amazed by.

Pam has tight hamstring muscles. After she has been running for several hours her right hamstring gets tight and starts to affect her gait. I have had good results giving her acupuncture treatments either before or after a long run. But no one had ever made a run like this before. (One man had run 265 + or - in the same way, and that is incredible as well.) So I was giving Pam a pre-run treatment and making arrangements to meet her and give massages to her when I asked her if we could try something different. EAR PELLETS. Auricular acupuncture is one way to extend a treatment and some people would say it enhances the effectiveness of any treatment. I like it, but do not always utilize it. I am now rethinking that approach.

I put two pellets (Silver coated stainless steel) into each ear. I was taught to use Shenmen (Neurogate) as an 'amplifier' with any other point. Then I found the most tender point near the hip joint/sciatic nerve area and placed a pellet there.

When I was riding with Pam she was saying how the 'ear seeds have made a huge difference.' Her gait was straight and her legs were tracking well. Two weeks after the run (she was out of town) we got together for another treatment and Pam told me "I am convinced those ear seeds made a complete difference in my run. My hamstring did not hurt for the entire run. In fact my hamstring did not hurt for two days after I removed the seeds and then only minimally." That is a HUGE difference.

I met her this Wednesday as she was preparing to go to London to run a marathon there and then return to Boston for their marathon. She wanted more seeds. It just goes to show…

\*\*\*

# A Story that **should** have been a BlogPost

# Wind in her face

When I first graduated from Southwest Acupuncture College I opened a clinic in Colorado Springs. One day I received a call from a patient telling me that she would be unable to come in for her appointment in two days, as she had had a stroke of Bell's Palsy affecting the right side of her face. I told her she was right, but she had to get on a bus and get down to my office as soon as she could!

When she came in, after a bit of convincing on my part, I saw what had happened and why she was so concerned. The entire right side of her face was drooping and would not respond to any muscular impulses, her right eye was closed and covered with gauze as it too would not close to blink.

In Oriental Medicine Bell's Palsy is seen as a "Wind Invasion" because of its sudden onset, usually without any warning that we are aware of. OM is pretty successful in treating this if the patient can get to his or her practitioner soon. The longer the "wind" is allowed to stay in one area the more challenging it is to extinguish.

I proceeded to give her the treatment, mainly involving face and scalp points, with some distal points on her hands and feet. After about 20 minutes or so I removed the gauze covering her right eye and told her to open and close her eyelid. She said she could not do that after the stroke. I said "Just humor me, OK?" She blinked her eye and said, Oh, My God!!! She was able to open, close and blink her eye intentionally and it blinked on its own as usual. She was completely amazed by this.

She came back daily for the next three days, then we returned to her regular weekly treatments. At that time you could not see any remaining signs of the Wind Invasion. After two weeks she returned to her neurologist for her follow up appointment. He looked at her and asked "What did you do to your face?" He could not believe that acupuncture had helped her, going so far as to tell her that whatever she had it must NOT have been a Bell's Palsy stroke, even though he was the one that diagnosed it in the first place.

I was very happy to have been able to help her in this way, and for a few moments was hopeful that I would be able to develop a working relationship with a local neurologist. This was the first time I had to learn that for some doctors even when they are confronted directly with the effective treatment of a condition, their preconceived opinions will outweigh the evidence they are seeing with their eyes and or electronic scanning devices.

I will still say that if you or someone you know has a stroke of Bell's Palsy get them to an acupuncturist as soon as possible. OM is also effective in treating a traditional stroke, though as you can imagine it is more challenging and Western Medicine is the first step. OM can integrate with WM in the treatment, but WM is the first and primary treatment in a traditional stroke condition.

# Chapter 13

# Balance and Perseverance

When you hear the word "balance" what comes to mind? For me, one thing I almost always think of is physical balance; I guess that is due to the many years I spent in the martial arts. But it does provide a good analogy as a way to explain my viewpoint.

When I am executing a jump-spinning back-side kick, balance is critical. I am literally about 2 ½ feet in the air and spinning like a top. At just the right instant my 'coiled up' kicking leg extends as fast as it can to impact the target. If I am out of balance I will very likely fall at some point in the process.

I had to work very hard, over a long time to develop a sense of awareness about my body and its balance. It is not like you can just jump up and perform these kinds of maneuvers effectively without practice, patience and perseverance.

The very same process can be used in learning about your own body. Well maybe you won't want to be practicing jump-spinning back-side kicks, but you get the idea. It is a matter of learning, practicing and persevering. If you knew how many times I fell on my face or other less glamorous parts of my anatomy while I was learning this kick, you would understand more about perseverance. When I would fall I would pick myself up, consider what happened and why it happened and then do it again, and again, and again.

Balance in our lives is all-inclusive.

We need to get enough exercise, but that needs to be balanced with enough rest. We need to eat enough, but not only does it need to be of a good quality we also need to allow time for our digestive tract to process and eliminate the foods we ate. We need to have times of mental activity as well as times of non-activity. Just watch a sunset and "veg out".

There are times when you are physically training your body when your mind will be 'on' but your body will not. You learn to relax with this; it is part of the process. Just as when your body is 'in the zone' but your mind may be out to lunch.

When you are learning to listen to the intrinsic rhythm and balance of your body there will be days when you are on target and integrating information exceptionally well; and there will be days when you just cannot seem to make heads or tails out of what your body is telling you. On days like that, you will need to persevere; just hang in there and do what you already know works for your body. Be sure to get enough sleep, good food and give yourself a break somewhere in the day.

I do want to encourage you to take the time to learn what your body is telling you. Your body can tell you so much more than we currently accept from it; we just have to learn to listen and accurately interpret what we are being told.

Here is an exercise for that. On one level it is exceedingly simple; do not let that fool you. It works when you get your mind 'out of the way' and listen to your body.

In your dominant hand hold something inert that weighs a couple of pounds. I use a rock or glass jar, because I do not know of anyone that is allergic to rocks or glass. I am sure there are people that are allergic to rocks or glass, but none that I know of. Anyway, hold this rock for about 30 seconds next to your belly button with your eyes closed, and then lift your hand holding the rock to about shoulder height. Gauge how hard that was to lift. Now, while still holding the rock in the same hand, pick up whatever it is that you are testing and hold that next to your belly button with your eyes closed for about 30 seconds. Now lift the rock again. Did it take more energy to lift the rock, or less energy? If it took "more energy" your body is telling you that substance is not good for you. If it took "less energy" your body is telling you that substance is good for you.

Here is my understanding of this. For example, let's say you are testing whether or not a potato is good for you. When you tune in to how much energy it took for you to lift just the rock you were setting a baseline. "It takes X-amount of energy for me to lift this rock today." When you held the potato next to your belly button the *"energetics"* of the potato had already entered into your being-ness. Then when you lifted the potato, it gave you a comparison to the baseline.

The trick is to listen to what your body is telling you.

There is a distinct difference between this and traditional muscle testing. The difference is that YOU are the only one involved in the testing. It is my belief that the perception of the person performing the muscle test will have an impact on the result of the test. It is like I am saying to myself as I am testing you "Oh I know this is good for you" and subconsciously pushing down with subtly less force than before. Or the opposite, saying "I know this is bad for you" and pushing down harder, even though I am consciously not aware of the change in force I am exerting.

So as simple as this test is, it can be used for foods, herbs, pharmaceuticals or anything you are going to ingest. (There are some very intelligent scientists that I respect that believe this can even be used to evaluate thoughts you have about yourself. Start with a "true statement {Your Name} and compare that to a "belief you have about yourself." Compare the results for yourself.) Again, I will say do not let the simplicity fool you.

If you take the time to test the foods you eat and are disciplined in your choices, you will be surprised at the foods you are currently eating that are not making you stronger. If you do this test and then implement what you learned and give your body two weeks you will probably be very surprised at how you are feeling, thinking and sleeping.

This is what I mean by balance; making small changes at a time to return to your natural state. For example if you drink a six-pack of beer a day on the weekend I would not tell you to quit drinking; rather I would say cut it down to four beers a day during the weekends for a month, then cut it to two beers a day on the weekend, then decide if you want to quit totally or what is right for *you*. This is all about listening to what our body is telling us and making corrections along the way.

By perseverance I mean making a choice to create a better state of health and then sticking to it. Doing whatever it takes to allow your body to return to its normal state of health, or at least as close as it can.

# Chapter 14

# The Spirits Within

Here I am going to talk about different aspects of who we are and how these aspects interact to form our consciousness. It is important to remember that when Oriental medicine was just starting the Ancients had not only a different world view, but their powers of observation were restricted to what they could see, touch, hear or smell. So in order to make a complete understanding of how we operate in the world the Ancients saw "Spirits" as integral to our humanness. The Ancients perceived that 'something' had to be "driving" us to act and interact in the curious ways that we do.

I think that what we conceive as 'Spirits' and what they conceived are significantly different.

First of all this was between 2-3,000 years BCE, so it was not in conflict with or in agreement with any currently recognized religion. This worldview predates all organized religion that I am aware of. I bring this up because I have had prospective patients ask me if Oriental Medicine is a "pagan belief system" or say that they have to talk with their pastor to see if it is OK to get acupuncture treatments. Of course I encouraged them to talk to their pastor about this, but I also attempted to express it has NOTHING to do with religion any more than a fish has to do with bicycle racing.

I think we could all agree that everyone has "Divine" aspects to their beingness. It is the huge amount of variation of their expression of the *Divine* that creates the discrepancies we experience in each person. In my opinion the statement that all men (and women) are created equal is a statement about our *Spiritual levels of Creation, or Divinity*; it is not truly an accurate statement of our physical reality.

There are several aspects to our Spirit as seen through Oriental medicine. The first one is the most common, though in my perspective it is the compilation of all of these aspects and worked with through our experience that becomes our true Spirit.

I will take some basic definitions from a great book and expand upon them. The book is *Rooted in Spirit* by Claude Larre, S.J. & Elisabeth Rochat de la Vallee (See Reference list in back) I appreciate their concise descriptions of these Spirits as seen in their glossary; any discrepancy in my descriptions is my own interpretation and should not be seen as a reflection on their fine work.

## SHEN

In Oriental Medicine the term "*Shen*" is used to express what we call "the Spirit", it is the part of ourselves that is responsible for mind/body/spirit integration, or "*MINDBODYSPIRIT.*" There is no true separation, though each can be addressed separately it is understood that what affects one will affect all.

*Shen* is the lightest, most insubstantial of all substances, and it is the most refined. *Shen* defines *Qi*, (our minds define the universe/reality). It is more refined and even less substantial than *Qi*.

*Shen* is the force that actively creates the manifestation of *Qi* (the body). If the "Spirit" did not want to create a physical body it would not have incarnated into the world. It is the "Will" of the *Shen* that is manifesting as a physical being in order to have the experiences that it needs to have in order to evolve on a Spiritual level. Everything that happens is part of this evolution, whether we see these experiences as 'good' or 'bad' is not the point.

*Shen* is the vitality behind Jing (Essence) and *Qi*, a loss of vitality is a *Shen* deficiency. A person with a strong *Shen* will be vital, vibrant and present in her or his world.

*Shen* helps to uphold the character of the body; when one is becoming 'defeated' it will be reflected in the way he or she carries him or herself in the world.

The *Shen* is the spirit that is stored in the Heart. This spirit is seen as the Guide, or the facility through which one sees and interacts with the world. Because of this it is said that "When the *Shen* is disturbed, people are crazy." We all know people who are "just a bit twisted (or more)" these individuals are reflecting a distortion in their *Shen*.

The source of *Shen* is primarily "Pre-heaven *Qi*", which is created by the process of reproduction, which is why it is so important for the parents to be to be in the right "head and Heart" space at the time of conception. The internal stresses that each parent has at the time of conception are a part of the mix that is added to the Spirit that is incarnating into the new fetus.

*Shen* is also acquired through life experiences. The myriad of our life experiences adds to, or subtracts from the strength of our *Shen*.

Traditionally it is said that the *Shen* is nourished by: food, water, and air and that all of these have to be of good quality and adequate quantity. I also feel that the *Shen* is nourished by our thoughts, feelings, actions and the company we keep. It is also very important to your *Shen* that you get sufficient rest, both sleep and just quiet time.

The functions of the *Shen* include guiding the BodyMind and directing the activities of *Qi*. If the *Shen* is twisted you can see how it will affect the quality of the state of mind of an individual. Maybe thinking of this analogy will clarify it for you; if a lens is distorted it cannot give a clear image to the viewer. In this analogy the *Shen* is the lens and if it is distorted it cannot give a clear accurate image to the viewer which would be your Inner-Divine-Godhead, or Soul.

A dysfunction within the *Shen* causes physical and or mental disease. Stated another way, if the *Shen* is distorted it can manifest as psycho-emotional disease and or as physical disease. Emotional problems, psychological and emotional shock, disturbances of psychological/mental nature are all reflections of disturbances of the *Shen*.

In the BodyMind the *Shen* appears in the Eyes, the sparkle of the eyes is the *Shen*. When that sparkle is disturbed, the *Shen* is disturbed. I am sure you have heard the expression that the "eyes are a window into the Soul." Be aware of and respectful of the image you see when you look into someone's eye, it is an accurate window into the state of their *Shen*.

There are many manifestations of disharmonies of *Shen* but the primary ones are a "muddled personality" (where one seems to be in a 'fog' no matter what their circumstances or physical health may be), and or forgetfulness and slow thinking. Other signs of a Shen disharmony are insomnia and or eyes that lack luster.

It is seen as a general Spirit disorder when a person experiences insanity, by which it is meant that it is more inclusive than just a *Shen* disturbance.

## HUN

The *Hun* are 'spiritual souls', or 'rational Spirits', also seen as the soul breath. These are earthly Spirits said to be animated by the same movement as the clouds.

The Earthly spirits are contraposed to the Heavenly Spirits (*Shen*). Their dwelling place in the body is the Liver. The *Hun* are an anchor to keep our *Shen* connected to the physical plane.

## YI (Intent)

The literal translation of *Yi* includes meaning, significance, intention, idea, opinion, and personal feeling. It also includes the intention of the Heart, what the thinking, speaking, and acting person puts into what he emits in sounds, thoughts or acts. Notice how thoughts are integral to this concept. It is vital to recognize that what one thinks has import in the world in which we live. Your thoughts do contribute to and create the reality in which we all live.

With various slight changes in the character the ideogram shifts its meaning though all are still "*Yi*";

*Yi*: to apply oneself (intent is seen as arising in the Heart); to remember, to recall one's spirit, to apply one's Heart and one's thought to something. It is the application of the Heart that takes into account what comes and presents itself. Again the inclusion of the Heart is seen to reflect the Spiritual aspect of the Heart.

*Yi*: A person's intent; a calm and peaceful atmosphere; the possibility of appreciating in a just way; to foresee exactly and to provide to each according to his need, indefinitely.

By appreciating each individual in such a way as to be able to provide just what they need may seem like enabling their co-dependence but I think there is a deeper way of interpreting this. What if you see that their need is to truly become independent? Would that not guide your actions to help their *Shen* grow and become independent?

*Yi*: the location of intent in the fleshly body is the chest, *the seat of intelligence*, of awareness, of feelings, and of personal opinions and viewpoints.

Note how the 'seat of intelligence' is NOT the brain or the 'mind' but is within the chest where the HEART is.

## PO

The *Po* are spirits that perceive through the senses; they are Spirits of the Earth which I take to mean they are substantive. They are the Corporeal Soul, the Soul of the fleshly body. The *Po* are mortal, they die with the physical carcass as contrasted to the *Shen* which is immortal. The *Po* are opposite to the Essences (*Jing*) that rise and disperse lightly in the body, charged with elements of vitality. At the time of death the *Po* evacuates the body through the perineum also called the 'gateway of Life & Death'. Their dwelling place in the body is the Lungs.

## JING

*Jing i*s the word used to describe the concept of "essence", specifically Kidney Essence. Along with *Qi* and *Shen*, it is considered one of the "Three Treasures" of Traditional Oriental Medicine.

*Jing* is stored in the Kidneys and is the most dense physical matter within the body (as opposed to *Shen* which is the lightest and most volatile). Jing is said to be the material basis for the physical body.

Production of semen, and menstrual blood, or pregnancy and childbirth, in the woman, are believed to place the biggest strains on *Jing*. Because of this, some even equate *Jing* with semen, but this is incomplete. *Jing* is the deepest physical manifestation of our beingness, but it is also an *energetic component* of our life experience.

One is said to be born with a set amount of *Jing* (also called *Yuan Qi*) and one also can acquire *Jing* from food and various forms of stimulation (correct exercise, study, meditation.) It is said that *Jing* is consumed continuously in life; by everyday stress, illness, substance abuse, sexual excess, etc. prenatal *Jing* by definition cannot be renewed, and it is said it is completely consumed upon dying.

### *Jing Qi* & *Jing Shen*

*Jing Qi* is the Essences and Breath that constitute the crucible wherein Life is created and maintained. The Essences (*Jing*) give themselves to the transformations in order to start up the Breaths (*Qi*). The breaths resulting from the transformations of the *Jing* are the *Qi* of the deep, authentic life of a being. Transformations are the effects of the *Qi* working on the *Jing*.

*Jing Shen* is the Vital Spirit, the animating Spirits of the *Jing*. It is human vitality at its most subtle level of expression. *Jing Shen* is the active totality of life, active for life's clear and conscious governance. The *Jing* fastens the *Shen* in place and give them a way to be expressed. The *Shen* is to free the subtlety of the *Jing* for the higher operations of Life.

# Chapter 15
# Women's Health

Now, as we all know women are complex creatures. This is true in every sense of the word. The good news is that Oriental Medicine is very effective in treating all phases of a woman's health. In fact I believe it is the most effective and least invasive form of medicine for a woman.

First of all let me outline the cycles of growth as understood by Oriental Medicine. The cycles are 8 years for men and 7 year cycles for women. These cycles are literally thousands of years old, and I do not think they remain as accurate as the rest of OM observations. In particular I do not think these cycles account for the improved nutrition we had up until the last generation, nor do they include the effects of radio waves, electromagnetic forces, chemicals, or stress in general.

The woman's cycles are as follows: at 7 yrs. of age her baby teeth are replaced by permanent ones, and her hair grows. At 14 yrs. of age the 'dew of heaven' arrives (menstruation), her periods become regular and she can conceive. At 21 yrs. the Kidney Essence peaks, her wisdom teeth come out and growth is its most luxuriant. At 28 yrs. her tendons and bones become strong, her hair grows its longest and her body is strong and flourishing. From the age of 35 years onward she slowly begins to lose radiance and health. At the age of 49 the 'dew of heaven' dries up (onset of menopause).

I find these cycles interesting, in particular the 7th cycle, 49 years old. Historically, worldwide a woman's average onset of menopause is 50.2 yrs. Pretty close I would say.

During my time as an acupuncturist I focused on treating all forms of women's health issues. This was partially a pragmatic decision in that women tend to listen to their bodies more and will come in for treatments. It was also due in part to my fascination with how well women's cycles seem to respond to acupuncture and herbology.

Oriental Medicine is very effective in regulating a woman's cycle so it is not problematic for her or her loved ones and co-workers. In general, regulating a woman's cycle is about two things: Building *Qi* & Blood, and Moving the *Qi* and Blood. If you have a problematic cycle and work with your acupuncturist you will probably be very amazed at the difference immediately, and in three full cycles things should be back to normal.

From the end of her menses a woman has to build *Qi* and blood for two weeks. I strongly recommend eating some red meat as there seems to be nothing like that for building blood. Two weeks after (at ovulation and after) she needs to change the focus to moving the *Qi* and blood.

For the first week after ovulation (the week before her period) it is really important to move the *Qi*. There are many ways to do this, but physical exercise is one of the best. Because a woman's *Qi* tends to get stagnant during this time she may tend to get angry. This can be greatly reduced by good healthy cardiovascular exercise. It will help a lot to get a good sweat in every day for as close to an hour as you can.

The week of her period it is not recommended to get that level of exercise, but still getting some exercise in will be a good idea. I would recommend yoga as it has many good postures to ease you through the moon time. Any reputable yoga teacher will tell you "No inverted postures during menstruation".

If you experience breast tenderness and distention the week before your period ask your acupuncturist about a *gwasha* treatment in the intercostal (the soft spaces between the ribs) from the middle of your side ribs back towards your spine. Let me explain this to you.

The Liver meridian comes up from your big toe to just under your breasts, on both sides. It is supposed to connect to the Lung meridian just above, in the pectoral muscles. If the breast tissue does not let the *Qi* flow smoothly you will experience the sensation of tenderness and distention. *Gwasha* is a technique so old as I know as far as I know no one knows who invented it, but it is scraping the oiled skin with a hard stone or spoon. *Gwasha* strongly moves *Qi* and blood. By performing *gwasha* from the middle of your side ribs towards your back you will be literally pulling the stuck *Qi* and blood out of your breasts and that will reduce or remove the tenderness and distention. A little oil on the skin and not too much pressure works best. I used to get my patient's to bring their partner's in so I could teach him or her how to do this. It is very simple and very effective.

Another very important issue to a woman is pregnancy and childbirth. These are both well suited for Oriental medicine. For now I will just say that if you are going to try to have a baby take a year before to get your body and Spirit in as good health as you can. I think of it like tending a field before you plant the seeds. You will not get as good of a crop if you just plant the seeds in a depleted field. The same is true for you in conceiving and raising a child. Do everything you can to ensure your body is as strong as it can be before you start this monumental undertaking.

And as my OB/GYN teacher taught us and I taught my students: **never yell at a pregnant woman!** That little one is receiving the energetic vibrations, be clear and calm when you address a mother-to-be.

Additionally after delivery of your child, Oriental Medicine is excellent at helping you restore your balance and vitality. The reality of postpartum depression is effectively reconciled through acupuncture and herbs. The herbal formulas will be totally safe if you are breast-feeding, which is highly recommended. Postpartum depression can be easily understood when you think of the amount of *Qi* and Blood the mother loses through childbirth. If you, or any of your friends or family are experiencing postpartum depression I strongly encourage you to seek out an acupuncturist/herbalist for effective treatments to resolve this condition.

The "Change of Life" does not have to be a roller-coaster ride. You actually start the process in your mid-thirties and the choices you make will have a profound effect on this major event in your life.

The first and most obvious place to start this discussion is to talk about birth control. One simple way to think of this is that males created birth control pills and do not have to experience the side effects of them. A birth control pill essentially fools your body into thinking you are pregnant. As the old TV commercials said, "It's not nice to fool Mother Nature."

Your body has a set number of eggs you are supposed to shed; if your body is thinking it is pregnant it is not going to slough off the lining in your uterus. If this continues for a long time your biological clock gets all cross-wired. On one level your body knows it is approaching menopause, but on another level you still have lots and lots of eggs to shed.

When menopause does come around can you see how this time will be even more complicated than it has to be? Your body would know that the "Dew of Heaven" is supposed to be drying up around this time, but your ovaries are still bearing eggs.

In my section on Men's Health I will get more deeply into this twist, but for now I will say: there are no known side effects of using a condom.

If you can keep your fully functioning regular cycle throughout your childbearing years it will pay off when it comes time to enter menopause. And even with that it may be a challenging ride but it will be smoother than if you have been tricking your body for the last 30 years.

# Men's Health

OK guys, it's our turn now. For starters, men are nowhere near as complicated as women mentally and emotionally. And the difference in the complexity of our bodies is even more pronounced.

The 8-year cycle for men is as follows: at the age of 8 years his Kidney energy is abundant, his hair and teeth grow. At the age of 16 his Kidney energy is even more abundant, the "Dew of Heaven" (sperm) arrives and he can produce a child (not to say we are ready to raise one!). At the age of 24 Kidney energy peaks, tendons and bones are strong, the wisdom teeth appear and growth is at its peak. At the age of 32 tendons and bones are their strongest, and the muscles are their strongest. At the age of 40, the Kidney is weakened the hair begins to fall out and the teeth become loose. As they say "It's all downhill after that…"

Again I want to emphasize that these cycles do not appear to be accurate at this time in our evolution. The cycles seem to me to be stretched both ways; by that I mean a girl will frequently start menstruation MUCH earlier than 14 and as we know boys are well into puberty (at least physically) before they are 16. But at the far end we are both much healthier as we age. But if you look you can still see wisdom in these cycles; so let's not completely throw them away.

Men need to find a balance between building *Qi* and Blood and moving it as well, but this does not have to be monitored as closely as a woman does. I think all men have a hormonal cycle as well.

It only makes sense for us to if you think about it. My experience has been confirmed by the men I have talked to.

Men have a six week cycle. I think it is easily tracked by what I would call 'levels of arousal." At the high point guys are seeing everything they are potentially attracted to, and at the low point we are not interested at all. Check it out for yourself, use a calendar and track your level for six months, then review it for patterns.

Now who said God does not have a sense of humor?

If my understanding of these cycles is correct and you are a heterosexual guy in a relationship, you and your partner will be at the same high point only three times a year. Of course you will also be at your low point three times a year as well. Try not to make any life-changing decisions when you are both at your low point…

But we still need to build *Qi* and Blood as well as move the *Qi* & Blood throughout our cycle, so talk with your acupuncturist about a good rotation of *Qi* and blood building and moving herbs and treatments. At least, we don't get cramps if we take the wrong herb at the wrong time of the month; your partner will.

While I am speaking of partners, I want to ask all the men that read this to consider their responsibility in the area of birth control. The only reason most men give for not using a condom is 'decreased sensitivity'. However I am asking you to consider the consequences that your partner may very well experience if you are asking her to use birth control pills. Her body *will* experience some side-effects, what they are cannot be determined beforehand, but as I mentioned when she goes through menopause she may have a much harsher experience of that than she would have if she had not been on the pill for years and or decades. I guess I am asking you to consider this from the angle of how much do you love your partner? Do you love her enough to not expose her to a chemical concoction that will have side effects, or is your physical experience all it is about?

Food for thought. But I will get off my soapbox now.

BlogPost: FRIDAY, JULY 28, 2006
## A student says something intriguing
Last night while teaching the Immunology class one of the students asked me if I had ever heard of the "Rife Microscope?" "No, what is it?" I asked. She said this inventor in the 20's or 30's created this microscope that allows one to see actual living cells, bacteria and viruses.
Google is such a handy little tool.... go to this web site: "www.navi.net/~rsc/rife1.htm" or the second one "www.navi.net/~rsc/rifebook.htm". It seems that this gentleman actually created a microscope that could see beyond the normally accepted range of magnification, and more importantly it could see the samples without killing them. Think about that for the treatment of disease. He did. In fact if one believes him he found and isolated one of the causative factors for cancer. Then he developed a non-invasive, non-traumatic way of treating the cancer. Even harder to believe, it worked. Oh my dear readers, I can hear you asking "What was the result, and why have we never heard of this?" Well that is a good question. I

can only tell you what little I read of his story before I got so excited I had to blog about it. (And I wanted to write something so you all know I am not freaked out about H5N1...) It seems that the good man was locked up for a number of years and the AMA worked hard to discredit his name and research. H'mm why does that NOT surprise me? OK, sorry I am getting too cynical.

Mr. Rife found a specific light frequency that would deactivate the malignant cells. Apparently it was not painful, or anything like that. The treatment would take 3 minutes every three days for about a week. The cancer was eradicated.

Now, think your way through this. This article (linked above) is saying that this treatment modality was effective at eradicating cancer. Yet none of us have ever heard of it. And the inventor was jailed and discredited. (This reminds me of the movie "The Count of Monte Cristo. It seems to be a good way of hiding or discrediting the want to know why this went down the way it did. It is a scary/sad/disheartening day when one thinks that there might have been an effective treatment for cancer in the 30's and we are still 'searching' for a cure 75 years later...

So, I found the comments of this student to be very interesting. She is a nurse and has seen enough of the allopathic medical model to be cynical in her own way. But for me it was really interesting because I have never heard of Mr. Rife or his universal microscope. I would encourage you to surf to the pages and see what you think. Of course, we all know that you cannot believe everything you read on the web, but that is the beauty of it. You have to be intelligent enough to discern the truth from the untruth. It's all there...

Till the next time.

# Chapter 16

# Internal Causes of "Dis-ease"

"The Five emotions can turn into Fire." What this is saying is that any one of the emotions, if unexpressed, or incorrectly expressed or exaggerated can stagnate the flow of Qi which will build, evolve and eventually turn into Fire. It is easy to understand when thinking of anger, but it can happen with any of the emotions, it just takes longer and maybe a more circuitous route. In these examples one of the primary diseases I think of is cancer. No, there has not been a definitive link established between the two, but I think of how my body responds when I have unexpressed anger or resentment, and then multiply and accelerate that 30 years and I can see how it could morph into cancer.

So let us revisit the External Causes of 'dis-ease': under normal circumstances, the weather will have no pathological effect on the body. The weather only becomes a cause of disease when the equilibrium between body and the environment breaks down. So no matter if you live in the heat of Phoenix or the damp of Miami, if your body's equilibrium is maintained by diet and exercise (at least) you will probably not have an environmentally caused disease.

However, there are other causes which are still "external." For example being born with a weak constitution will make it harder for your body to maintain that equilibrium. Also over exertion;

meaning physical or mental overwork. As I said earlier it is important to create time in your day to just let the brain rest; whatever you find to be the most relaxing. Personally I love to watch the city skyline at night and just breathe.

**Physical overwork** will also take a heavy toll on your body over time. Now I know it is important, and some jobs are harder physically than others, but after a couple of decades you need to consider moving up, or moving on.

**Excessive physical exercise** can also be very detrimental. I know that I have mentioned the importance of exercise several times, and I truly believe it is important. What I am talking here is finding the correct amount and type of exercise for your body at any given stage of life. For example I used to train really hard, 6 days a week for over 4 hours a day, sometimes 8 hours in a day. I would ride my bike to college, over 10 miles each way, then teach class at night. But that was nearly 15 years ago, now I am in a different stage in my life. I still love to train, but I do not push it as hard; I still ride my bike when I can, but not every day. What I am saying is my body is older, I have less energy to expend in exercise, but it is still critical for me to get exercise in as frequently as I can. I strive for at least an hour a day, six days a week.

Also in the list of areas to be aware of is: excessive sexual activity. As a younger person one has more energy to expend in this way, as we all know. But it is important to understand that this drains your Kidney energy and you only have so much Kidney energy to last your entire life; as my teachers always said: "Use it wisely."

The Ancients used to say that sexual activity had no consequence for women. I strongly disagree with this; I feel that statement is a reflection of the patriarchal society from whence it came. It does drain women, and we also have to be aware of their monthly cycle and if they have children, each of those factors is also draining to Kidney *Qi*.

Even in historical times **bad diet** was considered to be one of the external causes of disease. It is still true, plus we have the addition of chemicals, microwave cooking and foods that are pre-cooked and waiting on the shelf for you.

**Trauma** that is not properly resolved will lead to complications and diseases.

**Parasites and Poisons** are self-explanatory, though poison is becoming more insidious in our food chain.

And the worst in my opinion, whether from Western Medicine or Oriental Medicine would be: **wrong treatment**. This is when, for whatever reason the treatment you are given becomes the cause of disease. One clear example is our nation's overuse of antibiotics which is causing our bodies to be unable to defend against normal pathogens that are a part of our environment. Another example to consider is chemotherapy; one patient I had told me the chemotherapy he received for cancer would cause cancer at a later time according to his doctors.

Iatrogenic disease is in my opinion one of the sleeping giants under the rug that never, or rarely, gets talked about. Nonetheless approximately 250,000 deaths every year in the U.S. are directly related to diseases caused by medical treatments. This is the number 3 leading cause of death.

Do we need to discuss the irony of medical treatments being ON the list of leading causes of death, much less holding down a spot in the top three? Yes, I think we, as a society, do need to discuss this.

Internal Causes

Anger -- Makes Qi rise and affects the Liver. The term 'anger' should be very loosely interpreted to include resentment, repressed anger, irritability, frustration, rage, indignation, animosity and bitterness. Over a long time, it can cause Stagnation of Liver Qi or Blood, Rising Liver Yang, or Liver Fire. One of the most common symptoms caused by anger is a headache.

Joy -- Slows Qi down and affects the Heart. This term too must be broadly interpreted. Obviously, joy is not in itself a cause of disease. The Ancients would say "Joy makes the Mind peaceful and relaxed, it benefits the Nutritive and Defensive Qi and makes Qi relax and slow down." And "The Heart ... controls Joy, Joy injures the Heart, Fear counteracts Joy." What is meant here by 'joy' is obviously not a state of healthy contentment but one of excess excitement, which can injure the Heart. Our society lives in a state of continual overstimulation.

Worry and Pensiveness -- Knots the Qi and affects the Spleen. (Worry also affects the Lungs). Pensiveness means excessive thinking, excessive mental work or studying.

Sadness -- Dissolves Qi and affects the Lungs. Su Wen Chapter 39 says, "Sadness makes the Heart cramped and agitated, this pushes towards the lungs' lobes and the Upper Burner becomes obstructed, Nutritive and Defensive Qi cannot circulate freely, Heat accumulates and dissolves Qi."

Sadness leads to Lung-Qi Deficiency.

Fear- - Makes Qi descend and affects the Kidneys. The Su Wen says, "Fear depletes the Essence, it blocks the Upper Burner, which makes Qi descend to the Lower Burner." Fear and anxiety cause Kidney-Yin deficiency and rising of Empty-Heat within the Heart, a heat in the face, night sweats, palpitations and a dry mouth and throat.

Shock -- Scatters Qi and affects the Kidneys and Heart. (Mental or Psychic) shock suspends Qi, suddenly depleting Heart Qi. Historically it was said that "Shock affects the Heart depriving it of residence, the Mind has no shelter and cannot rest, so that Qi becomes chaotic."

BlogPost: WEDNESDAY, MAY 25, 2005
**Resentment ~ How it affects health.**
In an interesting series of events, I have been blessed with three patients that are all dealing with various issues of gall bladder dys-

function. Each patient is presenting with different 'issues' but have a similar underlying 'gall bladder issue.' Two of my patients have had their gall bladder removed; the other has avoided the knife so far. It is always interesting to me to see how allopathic medicine seems to like removing parts of our bodies. Now I know that sometimes it is required if the patient wants to survive, but it is also over utilized as an option that may not be required. I believe that an honest evaluation would agree with that observation. But, be that as it may.

In TCM I have read that if the Gall Bladder is involved, there are issues that the patient is holding on to or resenting. I have asked each of my patients if this is true and they have all said 'yes.' Of course we all have experiences that we wish would have turned out a different way, I know I have. The issue at hand is--can we let go of it and get past the emotions we are carrying from that experience? A different teacher from my past taught me that the meaning of the word resentment is to re-experience what we did not process at the initial time of the experience.

Think about that for a moment.

If I have a certain experience that I do not give myself permission to express my true emotion about, what happens to that emotion? I have read that the entire purpose of an emotion is to be expressed. That is not to say we should all be walking emotions. As with everything it is a matter of balance.

It is also true that our minds get addicted to the emotions we experience. Or as the saying goes: "Might as well face it. You're addicted to Love." Or in this case maybe the addiction is to resentment.

So back to my patients. What are the chances that acupuncture will help them with their experience of 'gall bladder' dysfunction? I honestly think that unless each one is willing and able to address and focus on the emotional content under the surface that acupuncture will only be a "Band-Aid" solution. That is not to say that it cannot help, but it is to say that the issue is not just the physical aspect and until the non-physical aspect is addressed (to some degree) the physical will continue to be a reminder to each of my patients. Stated in another way I am saying we each have to take responsibility for the consequences of the choices we have made. In these examples the choice seems to be to hold on to a past emotional experience and to let that affect their health. From a TCM perspective as well as an energy conservation perspective it seems much easier and healthier to just let it go.

I have told individuals that have 'hurt' me that the choice I have is to either forgive them, or forget that they have done that. I won't do both; if I forgive AND forget I set myself up to let that happen again. I do try to learn from my experiences and to not repeat the painful ones if I can help it.

I'll try to contemplate more and write more soon.

\*\*\*

# Chapter 17

# Closing Thoughts

I have tried to give a very brief overview of Oriental Medicine to help you understand the complexity as well as the potential depth of science within this fascinating medical field.

There are a couple of tremendously important areas of health that I have not entered into yet. The first is:

## Personal Accountability

In a society that seems to feel we are all entitled to nearly anything we want, I have to remind people about our own personal responsibility and accountability for our health.

We cannot afford to think that we are in a "welfare society" in which it is someone else's, or the government's responsibility for our health, or our health care. Each one of us makes choices every day that affect our health. Each one of us needs to accept the responsibility for making correct choices and to take the time and make the effort to learn how to make better choices for our health.

Think of how our society is opening up to the potential of "green jobs" or of a "greener environment." It is the same thing that we need to be aware of, and open up to, within the microcosm of our own body. As I heard the other day on NPR, we need to make scientific choices based on what is the best for a 12 year old girl; I understand this to mean that we need to look at the consequences of our choices in the light of what will those choices do to our bodies over the next 50-70 years.

Our society is being forced into grappling with huge issues at this time, ranging from worldwide economic complications, to global warming and the effects this is creating. We are also learning to look deeper within ourselves and our own unique set of internal values. I see a thread that runs through this all.

The thread I see starts with 'right thinking' and extends through 'right eating and right exercise.'

As that NPR story was suggesting if we learn to think of the consequences of our choices and how they would affect a young girl just entering into puberty over the long course of her life (or how it would affect our own health), it will give a different criteria for evaluating the decisions we make. This also reminds me of the ancient (though not current) Chinese and Native American philosophy of thinking about the implications of my choices and how they will affect seven generations. What will the outcome of these choices be for my great-great-great-great-great-great grandchildren? Will I want to eat foods that have chemicals that we know will affect my DNA? Will I want to be exposed to electromagnetic radiation on a continual basis? Will I want to deplete my body by over exercising, or conversely not keep my body in good health by not exercising at all?

I am not saying all technology is bad, far from that. I use and appreciate technology all the time. I am saying that we need to be aware of the consequences of our overuse and dependence on technology as well as the actual side effects of the use of technology. As a quick aside, are you aware that in Japan there are many, many areas where you cannot use a cell phone in public, because of the microwave radiation they emit? Think that through, considering the implied question of why is that not even making news in our country?

What I am attempting to convey is that each one of us has a myriad of choices before us at every moment of our lives, what we do with these choices will create consequences. The consequence of deferring the responsibility of making correct choices is one that is measured in our health. When we are younger the consequences do not seem that significant, yet as we age we see the consequence of each decision is like that snowball starting to roll down the mountainside. It started out fairly small, but it gathers speed and mass as it proceeds. When I was training and or teaching martial arts it was stated that "impact equals mass times acceleration." In the context of this discussion the impact (consequence) of a decision is a combination or multiplication of the initial significance (mass) of that decision times the acceleration (how long we have been doing this, and or how slippery of a slope one is trying to stand on).

So eating a meal of junk food is really no big deal. But this same diet over a period of years is a HUGE deal. Or stated another way a small mass times a great acceleration equals a huge impact.

## "Wellness-centered way of living."

This is my new interpretation of 'five-phase' theory.

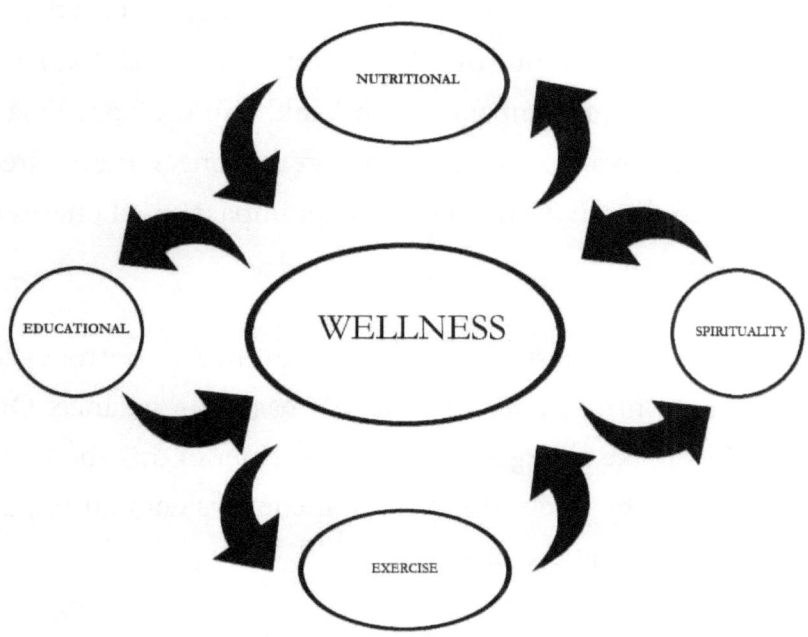

When I was discussing five-phase theory I had a diagram of a circle around a star to give a visual depiction of this theory. That is the most common, though not the only way of imaging a five-phase system. Another visual depiction would place *Earth* in the center and each of the remaining phases at polar opposition; top and bottom, left and right. In this depiction the energy travels from *Earth* to a particular phase and then returns to *Earth*. I see this as almost a four petal flower with a strong center.

I will place *WELLNESS* in the center position as I feel our health, on all levels and meanings, is the center-point of our life. Above *wellness* I place *NUTRITION*, as the fuel we put into our body has a direct impact on the wellness we experience. Below *wellness* I place *EXERCISE*, as the degree and amount of exercise has a distinct impact on our health. To the left I place *EDUCATION*, by which I mean not only direct traditional learning, but also the art of learning to listen to our own body and wisdom, as that has a critical and significant impact on our health. To the right I place *SPIRITUALITY*, because learning to have a stronger, more direct connection to the *Divine* has a significant impact on all phases of our health and wellness.

This model of five-phase theory does not utilize a 'control cycle' or a 'reverse-control cycle.' Instead it is based on balance. One could almost make an argument that the center of this should be labeled balance, but I do not think that conveys enough importance to the center phase of *Wellness*.

*Wellness is more than just the absence of disease*; it is a state of being that incorporates "thriving." Wellness is all-encompassing; it includes our physical, emotional, psychological and Spiritual being-ness When any one of these 'bodies' is out of balance it affects all of the others.

Each one of us has a significant, yet largely unrealized potential of power. It has been shown that when one person in a 'network' is happy and healthy it has a large, positive effect on the happiness and therefore the health of everyone in that network. So what this says is that when you are happy and healthy it does impact everyone in your network, whether that is work or family, or whether or not they even know of this does NOT seem to matter. It is transmitted throughout the network without direct communication about it. This communication is in effect whether or not one is happy or not, healthy or not. The unhappy, unhealthy individuals also have an effect on the entire network.

As each individual in a network has an effect on the overall status of that network, each one of us has an effect on our society as well. One could reasonably say that the reason our society is so 'whacked out' and out of touch is because so many of the individuals within society are 'whacked out' and out of touch.

I remember an interview with the Dali Lama where a reporter listed all of these serious conditions and situations in the world, and then asked the Dali Lama what he would do about them. The Dali Lama responded "I will work on myself." I am asking *you* to consider the truthful significance of that answer.

I would also remind you that as each one of us becomes more centered and balanced it will ripple out into our society. It is inconceivable to me that we could have a society of healthy, balanced individuals and have a society that is as out of balance and ill as our society currently is. Or as that old saying goes "As above, so below."

Now in fairness I have to acknowledge that facing these issues and making these types of changes in one's life is very challenging. There is no doubt about that; however if YOU really want to change things in your life who else is going to do it? Additionally I would add that if it were easy everyone would do it.

Albert Einstein once said, "Insanity is defined as doing the same thing in the same way and expecting different results." By that definition I would have to say our society is insane.

I would venture to say you initially picked up and read this book because on some level you are not satisfied with some aspects of your own health. While I have tried to explain how Oriental Medicine works, a bigger goal of mine is to help you to see the consequences of your choices. Again I go back to 'Right Thinking, Right Eating and Right Exercise'; these three areas are critical to your health, short term and long term. And as you consider these aspects of your life I hope you clearly see there is NO ONE ELSE that can do this for you.

Oriental Medicine can help so many aspects of one's health that I cannot even begin to list them all. OM is very powerful, though it is subtle. OM deals with 'root causes' of dis-ease. Emerging science is showing that what we think has a significant impact on our state of health.

Many times, readers of this type of book do so because on some level they are not satisfied with all aspects of their own health. In addition to explaining how Oriental Medicine works, a bigger goal of mine has been helping readers see the consequences of their choices. Again, I go back to 'Right Thinking, Right Eating and Right Exercise'; these three areas are critical to your health, short term and long term. And as you consider these different parts of your life, I hope you clearly see there is NO ONE ELSE who can do this for you.

Oriental Medicine can help so many aspects of one's health that

I cannot even begin to list them all. OM is very powerful, despite being subtle. OM deals with 'root causes' of dis-ease. Science is now showing that even our thoughts have a significant impact on our health, a field that is called Psychoneuroimmunology. The other scientific field of interest here is called Epigenetics, which is showing that the longer one lives the less significant DNA is and the more significant environment becomes. This is reflecting the importance of thought, diet, and exercise. Yet the traits developed from the environment do become a small part of what we leave for others to inherit.

What I am asking you to consider is your level of awareness about the consequences of your day-to-day decisions. It is these small, seemingly insignificant decisions that do cause significant change within your life experience.

One day in my martial training my instructor told us about the significance of a pendulum. He was saying how things are always changing, from 'this' to 'that.' He then explained how one side was not really any different than the other side; night is not better than day, hot is not better than cold, conservative is not better than liberal. What he said was imperative was to "ascend to a higher perspective." He then likened to these changes to an old grandfather clock with a pendulum swinging back and forth. He said the changes at the bottom of the pendulum were more pronounced or more drastic than the same changes experienced as one ascended and got higher on the pendulum.

I have since learned to equate this same perspective as "levels of consciousness." As one ascends the levels of consciousness one is 'closer to center' at all times and is able to see and appreciate from a higher perspective than one had in a lower level of consciousness.

One way of looking at this is to say that ascending the different levels of consciousness is *learning to listen to your body.* One has to be more centered, balanced and calm to effectively listen to his or her body. The analogy that comes to mind here is one of water in a bowl and looking at the reflection on the surface. If the water is agitated the reflection will be distorted, and if the water is full of dirt the reflection will not be clear. To accurately see the reflection within the bowl the water has to be clear and calm; or said another way to effectively listen to your body you have to have a calm mind and a clear Heart.

A Final BlogPost: THURSDAY, DECEMBER 24, 2009

## Harnessing the POWER of the INTELLIGENCE of the COMMUNITY

One of the things I have been trying to develop is a way to have an intelligent, rational discussion about health care in our society. I do not feel as the current national discussion is intelligent, rational or respectful. How can we expect to change this broken system if we are using broken thinking?

I want to start by addressing the inherent, yet hidden power of the innate intelligence of community. To do this I will relate a quick story from The Wisdom of Crowds by James Suroweicki. He opens his book with a story about the British anthropologist Francis Galton who was trying to prove how un-intelligent crowds were. What

Galton learned from this experiment flew directly in the face of what he had spent his lifetime trying to prove. To make a long story shorter, in 1906 Galton was at a fair and one of the competitions was to guess how much a cow would weigh after it was butchered and dressed. The competitors included butchers, farmers and average citizens. What Galton did that is of interest to me was to take the actual guesses by all the competitors and to find the average mean weight from that, then to compare that to the actual weight. The averaged guessed weight was 1,197 pounds, only one pound off from the actual weight of 1,198 pounds!

What this shows, if we read between the lines, is that the intelligence of ALL OF US is greater than the intelligence of any ONE of us.

This applies to my desire to have a discussion about health care because I am convinced that if we could actually generate a format where we could all put in our thoughts of how to create, monitor and fund a working health care system it would have the intelligence of our society; not just the biased intelligence of the special interest groups.

To create a format like this would require several things that I am aware of right off.

First of all in order to participate I feel one would have to agree to not attack anyone else's ideas or person. It does not matter about the quality of their idea; their idea will sink or swim on its own merit if we let it. But the idea one wants to attack may spark someone else to have an idea that sparks someone else to have a genuinely good idea. If we stop that process by attacking the idea or the person we ALL lose.

Secondly I feel we would need to agree that the system we have is broken.

My thinking is that if we can address health care and start to develop healthier individuals within the community it will spread out and these individuals will develop a healthier community in all areas; the environment, the economy, our schools and homes.

I also feel that if we can create this format in a functional manner we could use this model to discuss the environment and reap incredible rewards from that, as well as practical solutions to a most pressing issue. We could also then turn our focus to the Military-Industrial Complex and the Judicial-Industrial Complex.

My perception has been very strongly influenced by reading (and now re-reading immediately after finishing it the first time) "Spontaneous Evolution" by Bruce Lipton Ph.D. and Steve Bhaerman. This book is profound and I cannot find words to describe how enthusiastically I recommend it to everyone.

***

Respectfully,
Michael Clifford

# Recommended Reading List

*Eat Right 4 your Blood Type*, by Dr. Peter J. D'Adamo; G. P. Putnam & Sons.

*Healing with Whole Foods* by Paul Pitchford; North Atlantic Books.

*Wheat Belly Total Health* by William Davis MD; Rodale Books.

*Against All Grains* by Danielle Walker; Victory Belt Publishing.

*The Blood Sugar Solution 10-day Detox Diet* by Mark Hyman, MD; Little, Brown & Company Publishing.

*Primal Body, Primal Mind: Beyond the Paleo Diet for Total Health and a Longer Life* by Nora T. Gedgaudas CNS, CNT; Healing Arts Press.

*Prescriptions for Nutritional Healing* by James F. Balch M.D., & Phyllis A. Balch C,N,C.; Avery Publishing Group.

*Rooted in Spirit* by Claude Larre, S.J. & Elisabeth Rochat de la Vallee; Barrytown Limited Publishing.

*Magnificent Mind At Any Age* by Daniel G. Amen M.D.; Three Rivers Press

*Earthing: The most important health discovery ever?* By Clinton Ober, Stephen T. Sinatra M.D., & Martin Zucker; Basic Health Publications.

*Spontaneous Evolution: Our Positive Future (and a way to get*

*there from here)* by Bruce Lipton Ph.D. & Steve Bhaerman; Hay House Inc.

*Why Zebra's Don't Get Ulcers* by Robert M. Sapolsky Ph.D. Henry Holt and Company, LLC

*Introduction to Psychoneuroimmunology, Second Edition* by Jorge H. Daruna Academic Press, Elsevier Inc.


## My Three Favorite Herbal Supply Companies

(Alphabetical listing, not meant to compare)

- Evergreen Herbs
- Golden Flower Chinese Herbs
- Health Concerns

# Glossary

While I have attempted to be very clear in my use of certain terms I do understand that some of these words are new to many if not most of the readers of this book. Here I will give a simple explanation and a reference point to return to as you encounter unfamiliar words in the text of this book.

**Qi**: (pronounced "Chee" or "Key") Life-Force Energy, Vitality; all forms of life, whether plant or animal, have an indefinable form of energy within. There are no Western science tools that can detect the presence or absence of qi.

**Blood**: In TCM Blood is understood to be the vehicle that carries the qi throughout the body to nourish and sustain life; Blood is interwoven yet different than qi.

**Acupressure / Tui Na**: The traditional form of body work; may be used with acupuncture or as a separate effective treatment modality.

**Herbology**: The specific blending of traditional herbs used in various blends to address conditions within the context of TCM. NOTE: while there are valid concerns about the use of traditional herbs, if they are sourced correctly and used correctly TCM herbology is one of, if not the, safest form of medicinal treatments.

**TCM**: Traditional Chinese Medicine, also referred to in the book as Oriental Medicine (OM)

**Psychoneuroimmunology**: the Western science understanding that the "mind" has a definite, if as yet undefined, influence on the health of the body.

**Epigenetics**: A growing awareness that genetics itself can be influenced by the environment. It is now known that the genome will change in response to the needs of the organism and those changes will be passed down to the next generation. This means that your mother's early lifestyle influenced your genetic inheritance and your lifestyle will affect what your children inherit from you. You can learn about this emerging science by researching it on the web. It's controversial, so take time to draw your own conclusions.

**Diet**: All that one eats or drinks. The most powerful form of medicine or poison.

**Imbalances**: In TCM all health concerns can be understood in terms of imbalances; too much of one aspect, not enough of another aspect.

**Shen**: The Spirit within. All animal life has Shen, yet it is different within each specific individual. The Shen can be affected by the experiences and choices of one's life.

**Yin-Yang**: The inter-connected, yet opposing duality of life: hot-cold, day-night, male-female, good-bad. In TCM there are no things that are pure Yin or pure Yang; each is a blend of both with more of one aspect being more dominant.

*Acknowledgments*
*I would like to thank and acknowledge so many, many people that have contributed in one form or another to this book.*

*First of all, I wish to thank my teachers, both the formal teachers and the informal ones that came in the guise of being a patient or student. I have learned from all of you and I appreciate all of the myriad lessons and experiences each of you has taught me.*

*I would also like to thank my mother for all of her editing and suggestions of how to communicate the ideas presented in this book. Any lack of clarity, mis-communication, or inaccurate punctuation is entirely my own fault.*

*I am truly grateful to Bobby Sours for the images provided, he was able to take my bizarre ideas and translate them into workable images. Thank you, Sir.*

*The dragon image on the back cover comes from my brother-in-law, John Irick. He has created many fine metalwork images and has graced me with this fine guardian dragon.*

*This book would never have been published without the dedicated help of my technologically-proficient sister, Patricia Barlow-Irick.*

*I would also like to thank my wife, Mercedes for all that she does in my world.*

*Baraka-Bashad: May the Blessings Be.*

www.ingramcontent.com/pod-product-compliance
Lightning Source LLC
Chambersburg PA
CBHW020651220526
45464CB00001B/388